NCLEX-RN

made ridiculously simple

Andreas Carl, M.D., Ph.D.
Adjunct Assistant Professor
University of Nevada Reno
School of Medicine
Department of Physiology and Cell Biology
Reno, NV 89557-0046

MedMaster, Inc., Miami

D0793009

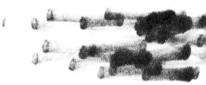

Notice: The author and publisher of this book have taken care to make certain that the recommendations for patient management and use of drugs are correct and compatible with the standards generally accepted at the time of publication. As new information becomes available, changes in treatment and use of drugs are inevitable. The reader is advised to carefully consult the instructions and information material included in the package insert of each drug or therapeutic agent before administration. The author and publisher disclaim any liability, loss, injury or damage incurred as a consequence, directly or indirectly, of the use and application of any of the contents of this book.

ISBN10# 1-935660-01-2
ISBN13# 978-1-935660-01-9

Made in the United States of America

Published by
MedMaster, Inc.
P.O. Box 640028
Miami, FL 33164

thanks to

Sharon Esguerra, RN
Michelle Villanueva, RN

"It may seem a strange principle to enunciate as the very first requirement in a Hospital that it should do the sick no harm."

Florence Nightingale, 1859

INTRODUCTION

The role of the nurse in the health care process is defined by the objectives of the entire health team – but you will find that the responsibilities of beginning nurses differ widely from one region of the US to another and from one facility to another. In addition health care is undergoing a major transition and the roles of nurses, physicians and physician assistants are constantly reassessed. For the beginning nurse it will be increasingly important to be as highly qualified as possible in order to take advantage of the many opportunities that arise in this new health care environment.

Nurses are involved in all aspects of health care and a thorough understanding of disease processes and the physiological as well as psychological needs of their clients are crucial for effective nursing care.

A major purpose of the NCLEX exam is to ensure <u>safe practices</u> by the beginning nurse.

YOUR CLIENT'S NEEDS:
➢ *Safe and effective care environment*
➢ *Physiological integrity*
➢ *Psychosocial integrity*
➢ *Health promotion and maintenance*

Between 60-75% of all questions on the NCLEX-RN deal with safe and effective care and the client's physiological needs. The remaining questions address the client's psychological needs, social needs and understanding of diseases and their prevention.

THE NURSING PROCESS:

The nursing process traditionally consists of 5 phases: Assessment, Analysis, Planning, Implementation and Evaluation. When studying for the NCLEX exam you need to pay particular attention to 3 of these 5 phases: **Assessment**, **Analysis** and **Implementation**. Much of *NCLEX-RN Made Ridiculously Simple* focuses on these three phases to make your study more effective, but this is not meant to imply that the other phases are less important. Development of a nursing plan and evaluation of whether the nursing goals have been achieved are a logical consequence of the nursing diagnosis. **Client Education**, which traditionally is part of the implementation phase has been given special emphasis in this book since you are expected to be able to teach your clients about disease processes, their likely outcomes and prevention.

iv

SOMETHING ABOUT CAT:

The NCLEX-RN is given as a **Computerized Adaptive Test (CAT)**. Each student receives a unique test because the computer selects the questions based on the student's prior answers. If you get an answer wrong, the computer will choose an easier question, if you get the answer right, the computer will select a more difficult question. You need to know that this is only a statistical process and you may find questions that are considered "difficult" easy, and questions that are considered "easy" more difficult; thus you probably will not be aware during the exam which direction the computer is going. The exam is terminated as soon as the computer reaches a statistical probability that you have passed or failed which will happen after a minimum of 75 and a maximum of 265 questions.

> ➤ **Minimum number of CAT questions: 75**
> ➤ **Maximum number of CAT question: 265**
> ➤ **Many candidates finish after just 75-100 questions.**
> ➤ **Very few candidates go all the way to 265 questions.**
> ➤ **CAT does not allow you to skip questions.**
>   *(If you don't know an answer just make your best guess and move on)*
> ➤ **CAT does not allow you to go back or change earlier questions.**
> ➤ **You can take as much time as you want for each question, however there is a maximum duration of 5 hours for the entire exam.**
> ➤ **Most candidates finish under 2 hours.**

Your success with the NCLEX exam not only depends on how hard you study, but also on what you study. Obviously, if you study what they ask, you will achieve a high score and will have little difficulty passing. I have prepared this book in order to help you maximize your efforts

WHY THE CHART FORMAT ?

I have arranged most material in this book in the form of charts. This allows for logical arrangement of NCLEX materials, which you can easily built upon and provides the maximum amount of information with the minimum amount of words for a lightning fast review.

Each page is a complete learning unit:
➤ Medical background information
➤ Side-by-side tables of easily confused facts
➤ The most pertinent facts of the nursing process
➤ Nursing tips and hints

This book is best used side by side with your other texts and review books. You may want to personalize the charts by adding any information that appears important or interesting to you. **The logical arrangement of nursing facts in charts will make it very easy to review all NCLEX subjects just a few weeks before the exam.**

You can – and should !!! – use this book as a TESTING TOOL in a similar fashion like you would study vocabulary of a foreign language: Cover the right part of the chart with your hand, and check if you can recall the key features or key associations of each item:

9.2.) SIGNS & SYMPTOMS

Kernig's sign	- **meningeal irritation** - patient supine, at first flex hip and knee ̶ ̶mpt to extend knee → pain or spasm occur
Brudzinski's sign	̶ on - ̶ ̶tly flex neck forward → ̶ knees occur
McBurney's sign	- app ̶ - rebo ̶ ̶ cBurney's point (1/3 fr ̶ ̶ o umbilicus)
Murphy's sign	- **acute cholec** ̶ - arrest of inspiratio ̶
Koplik's spots	- **measles** - small red spots wit ̶ ̶ ̶er on buccal mucosa - generalized rash will follow in 1-2 days

"Praying hands" borrowed from Albrecht Dürer.

vi

HOW TO PRACTICE MULTIPLE CHOICE QUESTIONS?

Practice as many questions as possible from (3), (5), (6) or any of the numerous other collections that are available. Regular practice will get you used to the testing situation and gives you a good idea about areas of strengths and weaknesses.

Don't use questions to "test" yourself. Don't be concerned about how many percent you get right. Mark all questions you get wrong with a pen, identify your areas of weakness and concentrate your studies on these. Later review just the questions you got wrong the first time and see how much you have learned. Or make a list of the items you answered wrong, and then read over this list the day before the exam to refresh your memory.

SYMBOLS

Tips and Hints
◊ Client Symptoms
● Client Signs

VISIT OUR WEBSITE
www.nclex-rn.net

THANKS

I wish to thank Michelle Villanueva, RN for her reading of the manuscript and help and excellent advice, S. Goldberg for providing the cartoons and Brian Foote for some illustrations.

RECOMMENDED TEXT BOOK

1. *Medical-Surgical Nursing: Assessment and Management of Clinical Problems*, Lewis et al., Mosby

POPULAR REVIEW BOOKS FOR THE NCLEX

There are many comprehensive review books for the NCLEX-RN available, and you should choose whatever fits best your own learning style:

1. *Mosby's Comprehensive Review of Nursing for NCLEX-RN*, Saxton et al., Mosby
2. *Mosby's Review Questions for the NCLEX-RN*, Nugent et al., Mosby
3. *Kaplan NCLEX-RN: Strategies, Practice, and Review*, Irwin, Kaplan Publishing
4. *Saunders Comprehensive Review for the NCLEX-RN*, Silvestri, Saunders
5. *Saunders Q & A Review for the NCLEX-RN Examination*, Silvestri, Saunders

Visit www.nclex-rn.net for more info.

FREE DOWNLOAD

Before you do anything else, please download a 1,000 QUESTIONS QUIZ for the NCLEX here:

www.medmaster.net

1,000 QUESTIONS QUIZ is in "mix-and-match style" and tied to the content of this book. Our "mix-and-match" style allows you to test several items at once in a much shorter time than the regular single-item practice questions you are familiar with.

You probably will find these questions difficult and challenging. Once you have worked with this book for a while, it will get easier and you will find that you have learned a lot.

IMAGE LINKS require a hookup to the Internet. You will find the most important and relevant images for the NCLEX exam here. Many times a picture says more than thousand words. Please try them all!

CONTENTS

PART 1: MEDICAL / SURGICAL NURSING
1. General Nursing Practices 1
2. Nutrition & Calculations 15
3. Fluids & Electrolytes 27
4. Cardiovascular Diseases 41
5. Respiratory Diseases 71
6. Gastrointestinal Diseases 89
7. Urogenital Diseases 123
8. Sexually Transmitted Diseases 137
9. Infectious Diseases 143
10. Diseases of the Blood 149
11. Endocrine Diseases 165
12. Musculoskeletal Diseases 181
13. Diseases of the Nervous System 195
14. Diseases of the Eyes & Ears 213
15. Diseases of the Skin 223
16. Injury & Poisoning 231

PART 2: CHILDBEARING & WOMEN'S HEALTH
17. Female Reproductive System 257
18. Maternity 273

PART 3: PEDIATRIC NURSING
19. Growth & Development 293
20. The Neonate 301
21. Infants & Toddlers 319

PART 4: MENTAL HEALTH NURSING
22. Psychiatry 339

PART 5: APPENDIX
23. Nursing Pharmacology 355
24. Conversions 377

ABBREVIATIONS 383

INDEX 385

PART 1: MEDICAL / SURGICAL NURSING

GENERAL NURSING PRACTICES

1.1. Good things to say
1.2. Bad things to say
1.3. The nursing process
1.4. Nursing diagnoses
1.5. Client's needs
1.6. Universal precautions
1.7. Proper position of client

1.8. Cancer screening guide
1.9. Patients with cancer
1.10. Vital Signs
1.11. Preoperative care
1.12. Postoperative care
1.13. Wound care

NUTRITION & CALCULATIONS

NUTRITION

2.1. Health promotion
2.2. Low-protein diet
2.3. High-protein diet
2.4. Low-cholesterol diet
2.5. Low-fat diet
2.6. Diabetic diet

2.7. Bland diet
2.8. Low-sodium diet
2.9. High-potassium diet
2.10. Other diets
2.11. Vitamins

CALCULATIONS

2.12. Dosage calculations
2.13. IV calculations

FLUIDS & ELECTROLYTES

3.1. Diffusion & Osmosis
3.2. Acid/Base physiology
3.3. Acid/Base disorders
3.4. Respiratory acidosis
3.5. Metabolic acidosis
3.6. Respiratory alkalosis
3.7. Metabolic alkalosis
3.8. Sodium levels
3.9. Simple dehydration

3.10. Overhydration
3.11. Potassium levels
3.12. Hyperkalemia
3.13. Hypokalemia
3.14. Calcium levels
3.15. Hypercalcemia
3.16. Hypocalcemia
3.17. IV solutions

CARDIOVASCULAR DISEASES

4.1. Physiology
4.2. Signs & Symptoms
4.3. Hypertension
4.4. Coronary heart disease
4.5. Chest pain
4.6. Other causes of chest pain
4.7. Angina pectoris
4.8. Myocardial infarction
4.9. Complications of MI
4.10. Arrhythmias
4.11. Pacemakers
4.12. Congestive heart failure
4.13. Assessment: Heart failure
4.14. Assessment: Shock

4.15. Hypovolemic shock
4.16. Pericarditis
4.17. Cardiac tamponade
4.18. Myocarditis
4.19. Rheumatic heart disease
4.20. Heart valves
4.21. Cardiomyopathy
4.22. Endocarditis
4.23. Blood vessels
4.24. Arteriosclerosis
4.25. Raynaud's disease
4.26. Aneurysms
4.27. Vasculitis
4.28. Phlebothrombosis

RESPIRATORY DISEASES

5.1. Physiology
5.2. Breathing patterns
5.3. Lung sounds
5.4. Pulmonary care principles
5.5. Pneumothorax
5.6. Upper respiratory infections
5.7. Pneumonia
5.8. Tuberculosis

5.9. Chronic obstructive pulmonary disease
5.10. Chronic bronchitis
5.11. Emphysema
5.12. Asthma
5.13. Restrictive lung diseases
5.14. Shock lung (ARDS)
5.15. Lung cancer

GASTROINTESTINAL DISEASES

6.1. Alteration in nutrition
6.2. Mouth: Signs & Symptoms
6.3. GI bleeding
6.4. Upper abdominal pain
6.5. Esophagitis
6.6. Hiatal hernia
6.7. Esophageal varices
6.8. Gastritis
6.9. Peptic ulcer disease
6.10. Liver: Signs & Symptoms
6.11. Liver: Lab data
6.12. Jaundice
6.13. Drug induced liver disease
6.14. Liver cirrhosis

6.15. Hepatitis
6.16. Gallbladder
6.17. Cholecystitis
6.18. Pancreatitis
6.19. Maldigestion
6.20. Diarrhea
6.21. Lower abdominal pain
6.22. Appendicitis
6.23. Diverticulitis
6.24. Hemorrhoids
6.25. Inflammatory bowel disease
6.26. Intestinal obstruction
6.27. Peritonitis
6.28. Colorectal cancer

UROGENITAL DISEASES

7.1. Physiology
7.2. Assessment: Urine
7.3. Lower urinary tract infections
7.4. Kidney stones
7.5. Kidneys: Lab data
7.6. Glomerulonephritis

7.7. Acute renal failure
7.8. Chronic renal failure
7.9. Kidney transplantation
7.10. Prostate hypertrophy
7.11. Prostate cancer

SEXUALLY TRANSMITTED DISEASES

8.1. STDS
8.2. AIDS
8.3. AIDS: Signs & Symptoms

INFECTIOUS DISEASES

9.1. Key list
9.2. Signs & Symptoms

9.3. Defense mechanisms
9.4. Nosocomial infections

DISEASES OF THE BLOOD

10.1. Blood
10.2. Blood cells
10.3. Red blood cells
10.4. Anemias
10.5. Blood products
10.6. Transfusion reactions
10.7. Acute leukemia

10.8. Chronic leukemia
10.9. Multiple myeloma
10.10. Lymphoma
10.11. Bleeding disorders
10.12. Thrombocytopenia
10.13. Hemophilia
10.14. DIC

ENDOCRINE DISEASES

11.1. Physiology
11.2. Pituitary hypofunction
11.3. Pituitary hyperfunction
11.4. Acromegaly
11.5. Cushing's disease
11.6. Conn's syndrome
11.7. Addison's disease

11.8. Addisonian crisis
11.9. Hyperthyroidism
11.10. Hypothyroidism
11.11. Diabetes mellitus
11.12. Insulin
11.13. Sulfonylureas
11.14. Metabolic Syndrome

MUSCULOSKELETAL DISEASES

12.1. Signs & Symptoms
12.2. Assessment: Arthritis
12.3. Osteoarthritis
12.4. Rheumatoid arthritis
12.5. Gout
12.6. Spondyloarthropathies
12.7. Systemic lupus erythematosus

12.8. Osteoporosis
12.9. Herniated disk
12.10. Carpal tunnel syndrome
12.11. Osteomyelitis
12.12. Leg amputation
12.13. Crutches & Canes

DISEASES OF THE NERVOUS SYSTEM

13.1. Signs & Symptoms
13.2. Glasgow coma scale
13.3. Central nervous system
13.4. Autonomic nervous system
13.5. Cranial nerves
13.6. Sleep disorders
13.7. Headache
13.8. Increased intracranial pressure
13.9. Meningitis

13.10. Stroke
13.11. Paraplegia / Quadriplegia
13.12. Peripheral neuropathies
13.13. Parkinson's disease
13.14. Multiple sclerosis
13.15. Amyotrophic lateral sclerosis
13.16. Bell's palsy
13.17. Epilepsy

DISEASES OF THE EYES & EARS

14.1. Refraction
14.2. Cataract
14.3. Blindness
14.4. Conjunctivitis
14.5. Chalazion & Stye
14.6. Glaucoma

14.7. Retina detachment
14.8. Assessment: ears
14.9. Otosclerosis
14.10. Presbyacusis
14.11. Ménière's disease

DISEASES OF THE SKIN

15.1. Skin lesions
15.2. Dermatitis
15.3. Acne
15.4. Seborrheic eczema

15.5. Psoriasis
15.6. Stasis dermatitis
15.7. Varicose veins
15.8. Skin tumors

INJURY & POISONING

16.1. ABC of trauma
16.2. Poisoning
16.3. Head trauma
16.4. Chest trauma
16.5. Abdominal trauma
16.6. Genitourinary trauma
16.7. Fractures
16.8. Sprains

16.9. Nerve injuries
16.10. Casts
16.11. Traction
16.12. Burns
16.13. Drowning
16.14. Altitude sickness
16.15. Bites & Stings

PART 2: CHILDBEARING & WOMEN'S HEALTH

FEMALE REPRODUCTIVE SYSTEM

17.1. Menstrual cycle
17.2. Contraception
17.3. Infertility
17.4. Menstruation
17.5. Primary amenorrhea
17.6. Secondary amenorrhea
17.7. Dysmenorrhea
17.8. Endometriosis
17.9. Pelvic inflammatory disease

17.10. Menopause
17.11. Nipple discharge
17.12. Fibrocystic change
17.13. Breast cancer
17.14. Breast self-exam
17.15. Cervical cancer
17.16. Ovarian cancer
17.17. Endometrial cancer
17.18. Uterine myomas

MATERNITY

18.1. Parity
18.2. Pregnancy: Signs & Symptoms
18.3. Pregnancy: Common problems
18.4. Pregnancy: Signs of danger
18.5. First trimester
18.6. Second trimester
18.7. Third trimester
18.8. Preeclampsia
18.9. The fetus
18.10. Fetal evaluation
18.11. Fetal heart rate
18.12. Assessment: Labor

18.13. Labor: First stage
18.14. Labor: Second stage
18.15. Labor: Third stage
18.16. Spontaneous abortion
18.17. Premature labor
18.18. Cesarean section
18.19. Abruptio placentae
18.20. Prolapsed cord
18.21. Postpartum hemorrhage
18.22. Puerperal infection
18.23. Mastitis

PART 3: PEDIATRIC NURSING

GROWTH & DEVELOPMENT

19.1. Nutrition
19.2. Motor development
19.3. Psychological development
19.4. IQ tests
19.5. Failure to thrive
19.6. Child abuse

THE NEONATE

20.1. Birth trauma
20.2. Apgar score
20.3. Vital Signs
20.4. Reflexes
20.5. Small & large infants
20.6. Prematurity
20.7. Postmaturity
20.8. Respiratory distress syndrome
20.9. Neonatal jaundice
20.10. Neonatal sepsis
20.11. Teratogens
20.12. Multifactorial birth defects
20.13. Heart defects: What to expect
20.14. Cerebral palsy
20.15. Down's syndrome
20.16. Esophageal atresia
20.17. Hypertrophic pyloric stenosis
20.18. Intussusception
20.19. Hirschsprung's disease
20.20. Congenital hip dysplasia

INFANTS & TODDLERS

21.1. The ill child
21.2. Proper position
21.3. Diaper dermatitis
21.4. Cryptorchidism
21.5. Infectious diseases of childhood
21.6. Incubation periods
21.7. Immunization schedule
21.8. Respiratory tract infections
21.9. Croup
21.10. Epiglottitis
21.11. Otitis media
21.12. Tonsillitis
21.13. Reye's syndrome
21.14. Rheumatic fever
21.15. Juvenile rheumatoid arthritis
21.16. Cystic fibrosis
21.17. Leukemia
21.18. Wilms' tumor
21.19. Febrile seizures
21.20. Enuresis
21.21. ADHD

PART 4: MENTAL HEALTH NURSING

PSYCHIATRY

22.1. The "difficult" client
22.2. Defense mechanisms
22.3. Signs & Symptoms
22.4. Mental status
22.5. Delirium & Dementia
22.6. Alzheimer's disease
22.7. Dementia & Depression
22.8. Grief & Depression

22.9. Personality disorders
22.10. Anxiety disorders
22.11. Hypochondriasis & Malingering
22.12. Major depression
22.13. Bipolar disorder
22.14. Schizophrenia
22.15. Drug abuse
22.16. Eating disorders

PART 5: APPENDIX

NURSING PHARMACOLOGY

23.1. Some trademarks
23.2. Famous side effects
23.3. Antibiotics
23.4. Nonsteroidal antiinflammatory drugs
23.5. Corticosteroids
23.6. Antihypertensive drugs
23.7. Nitrates
23.8. Diuretics
23.9. Congestive heart failure
23.10. Anticoagulants
23.11. Antiarrhythmic drugs

23.12. Asthma
23.13. Peptic ulcers
23.14. Sex-hormones
23.15. Drugs used in obstetrics
23.16. Anxiolytic drugs
23.17. Hypnotic drugs
23.18. Antidepressants
23.19. Lithium
23.20. Neuroleptics
23.21. Parkinson's disease
23.22. Chemotherapy

CONVERSIONS

24.1. Metric system
24.2. Apothecary system
24.3. Household system
24.4. Temperature conversion
24.5. Prescriptions

ABBREVIATIONS

INDEX

GENERAL NURSING
PRACTICES

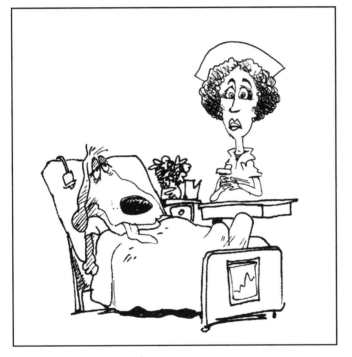

"Nurse, may I have the tree please…"

1.1.) GOOD THINGS TO SAY

broad opening	"How are things going today?"
clarify	"What does this mean to you?"
restate	"What you are saying is…"
acknowledge	"I see how upset you are about this."
empathy	"You seem sad today."
silence	*Show nonverbal interest!*

<u>Communication skills</u>:
➤ Express empathy
➤ Remain genuine and nonjudgmental
➤ Don't appear rushed
➤ Express sensitivity to client's culture and values

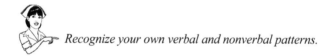 *Recognize your own verbal and nonverbal patterns.*

1.2.) BAD THINGS TO SAY

false reassurance	"Don't worry, everything will be all right."
belittling	"Don't be concerned, everyone feels like that."
judging	"It's your own mistake; if you had stopped smoking…"
defending	"We never make mistakes."

<u>Communication blocks</u>:
➤ Failure to listen
➤ Stereotypes and prejudice
➤ Cultural misunderstandings
➤ Language inappropriate for nurse/client relationship

1.3.) THE NURSING PROCESS

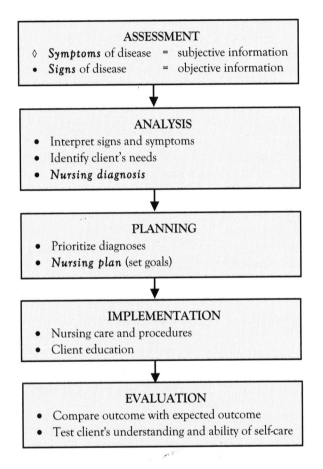

ASSESSMENT
- ◊ *Symptoms* of disease = subjective information
- • *Signs* of disease = objective information

↓

ANALYSIS
- • Interpret signs and symptoms
- • Identify client's needs
- • *Nursing diagnosis*

↓

PLANNING
- • Prioritize diagnoses
- • *Nursing plan* (set goals)

↓

IMPLEMENTATION
- • Nursing care and procedures
- • Client education

↓

EVALUATION
- • Compare outcome with expected outcome
- • Test client's understanding and ability of self-care

When studying for the NCLEX exam you may want to pay most attention to 3 of these 5 phases: **Assessment, Analysis** *and* **Implementation.**

1.4.) NURSING DIAGNOSES
(NANDA = North American Nursing Diagnosis Association)

➤ The nursing diagnosis is a statement of patient's problems and provides the basis for nursing care.
➤ Nursing diagnoses are health conditions that nurses are legally licensed to treat!
➤ Each nursing diagnosis is associated with several possible medical diagnoses!

NURSING DIAGNOSIS	MEDICAL DIAGNOSIS
= patient's condition (physio-, psychological, social)	= disease entity
EXAMPLES: - ineffective breathing pattern - fluid volume deficit - ineffective coping - knowledge deficit	EXAMPLES: - pneumonia - shock - major depression

-----Following are some of the most common NANDA approved diagnoses-----

A) PHYSIOLOGICAL:

NURSING DIAGNOSIS	TYPICAL NURSING INTERVENTIONS:
Impaired skin integrity	- change client's position every 2 hours - protect bony prominences with foam pad - massage to increase circulation
Fluid volume deficit	- measure intake/output, monitor electrolyte levels - encourage client to drink frequently
Decreased cardiac output	- monitor vital signs, assess for hypoxia or shock - weigh patient daily to detect fluid retention
Alteration in tissue perfusion	- monitor vital signs, respiratory rate, ECG, ABGs - monitor consciousness and neurologic status - monitor renal function

4

NURSING DIAGNOSIS	TYPICAL NURSING INTERVENTIONS:
Ineffective airway clearance	- place client in Fowler's position - postural drainage, percussion every 4 hours
Ineffective breathing pattern	- assess chest pain frequently, medication as needed - deep-breathe every 4 hours to prevent atelectasis
Impaired gas exchange	- monitor vital signs, ABGs, hemoglobin, hematocrit - check urine/stool for signs of internal bleeding
Alteration in bowel elimination: *Constipation*	- increase fluid and fiber intake - avoid use of bed pan - teach client to avoid habitual use of laxatives
Alteration in bowel elimination: *Diarrhea*	- fluid and electrolyte replacement - assess for signs of dehydration
Alteration in urinary elimination	- catheterization: only if necessary [1] - Kegel exercises to strengthen sphincter control

[1] *intermittent use helps to maintain integrity of bladder function.*

B) PSYCHOLOGICAL:

NURSING DIAGNOSIS	TYPICAL NURSING INTERVENTIONS:
Fear, Anxiety	- encourage client to express fears and emotions - assign same nurse to care for client if possible - involve client in planning care → sense of control
Dysfunctional grieving	- encourage client to express sadness and anger - encourage client and family to reminisce
Ineffective coping	- encourage emotional support: family, support groups - let clients increase self-care levels at their own pace

5

NURSING DIAGNOSIS	TYPICAL NURSING INTERVENTIONS:
Sensory-perceptual excess	- accept client's hallucinations or delusions (*do not challenge or ridicule!*)
Sensory-perceptual deficit	- compensate for loss of hearing, vision etc. by increasing other sensory stimuli
Alteration in thought process related to memory loss	- orient client to reality (sights, sounds): call client by name; mention place, time and date frequently - make family provide client with favorite belongings or photos to promote a sense of continuity
Potential for violence	- remain calm and unhurried → reduce client's feeling of lack of control - remove sharp objects, glass etc. - allow client to express emotions in non-violent way

C) SOCIAL:

NURSING DIAGNOSIS	TYPICAL NURSING INTERVENTIONS:
Social isolation	- spend time with client → increase trust - encourage group activities
Impaired verbal communication	- speak slowly and clearly in a normal tone - reduce client's frustration: Allow plenty of time for response - ask simple questions that require 'yes' or 'no' for an answer - *do not pretend to understand if you don't !*

6

1.5.) CLIENT'S NEEDS

MASLOW'S HIERARCHY OF NEEDS:
"Higher levels can only be achieved when lower needs are fulfilled."

self-actualization	fully achieving one's potential
self-esteem	confidence, usefulness and sense of purpose
love and belonging	need for affectionate relationships overcoming feelings of alienation and aloneness
safety and security	includes both physical and psychological safety
physiological needs	food, fluids, sleep homeostasis

*This hierarchy is important when formulating a nursing plan **(Planning stage)** to prioritize your care! Nursing care is mainly, but not exclusively, concerned with the client's most basic physiological needs and safety needs. But even "chronic low self-esteem" and "potential for enhanced spiritual well-being" are valid NANDA approved nursing diagnoses.*

7

1.6.) UNDERSTAND PRECAUTIONS

Standard precautions used for all clients regardless of diagnosis

gloves	**required whenever contact with <u>body fluids</u> is likely:** - blood - secretions, excretions - mucous membranes - non-intact skin *not required when simply touching intact skin*
gown	**required if <u>soiling</u> is likely**
mask	**required if <u>splashes</u> of blood or body fluids are likely**
hand washing	**<u>always</u> required, whether gloves are worn or not** - wash <u>before and after</u> contact with clients - wash immediately after gloves are removed - wash before touching non-contaminated surface or item
other precautions	- never recap used needles - discard needles in special "sharp container" - discard items contaminated with body fluids in a "biohazard container"

Universal precautions are also appropriate for patients with AIDS and patients with hepatitis B.

- For patients with hepatitis A additional contact precaution are required.

- For patients with tuberculosis and other serious respiratory infections airborne precautions (against droplets) are necessary.

1.7.) PROPER POSITION OF CLIENT

upine	head of bed flat client lies on back	spinal cord injury
rone	head of bed flat client lies on abdomen	after lumbar puncture for 3 h.
emi-Fowler's	head of bed elevated 30°	head injury increased intracranial pressure
owler's	head of bed elevated 45°	after cranial surgery bleeding esophageal varices dyspnea (cardiac causes)
igh Fowler's	head of bed elevated 90°	orthopnea status asthmaticus pneumothorax
endelenburg	head and body are lowered feet are elevated	shock
ims' semiprone)	lying on side	unconscious client (unless on respirator)

Most newborn babies should sleep in the supine position to reduce risk of SIDS: sudden infant death syndrome!

1.8.) CANCER SCREENING GUIDE

WOMEN:

	age	frequency
breast exam	> 40 years	yearly
mammography	> 50 years	every 1~2 years
Pap smear	all sexually active women	every 2 years

MEN:

	age	frequency
prostate PSA	> 50 years	yearly

MEN & WOMEN:

	age	frequency
digital rectal exam	> 40 years	yearly
sigmoidoscopy	> 50 years	every 3 years

1.9.) PATENTS WITH CANCER

➢ TNM: T=Tumor size, N=Lymph node status, M=Metastases

	NURSING INTERVENTION
chemotherapy	<ul><li>wear latex gloves, don't eat or drink when administering drugs (to prevent self exposure)</li><li>encourage good oral hygiene</li><li>monitor for **signs of infection** (highest risk 7~14 days after administration)</li><li>monitor intake / output</li><li>risk of bleeding: avoid aspirin</li></ul>
radiotherapy	<ul><li>antiemetic before treatment</li><li>provide good skin care</li><li>wash with water, avoid lotions and sunlight</li><li>**abdomen**: expect diarrhea or constipation</li><li>**upper body**: expect dry mouth (give plenty of fluids)</li></ul>
internal radiotherapy (cesium sticks)	<ul><li>bed rest during treatment (24~72 hours)</li><li>Foley catheter required</li><li>minimize time at bedside</li><li>if radiation source falls out: **do not touch!** (use forceps to put into lead container)</li></ul> CLIENT EDUCATION: <ul><li>don't touch source of radiation</li><li>call immediately if it dislodges</li></ul>

REVERSE ISOLATION TECHNIQUE:
(for example during bone marrow suppression)
1. Private room, laminar air-flow, sterile linen, sterile hygiene equipment
2. Put on shoe covers, put on mask and cap, put on sterile gown, gloves
3. Remove gown <u>after</u> leaving room

1.10.) VITAL SIGNS

temperature oral 37°C = 98.6°F	- for routine oral is sufficient - rectal is more accurate than oral (0.4°C or 0.8°F higher than oral)
pulse 60~80 per minute	- count for 30 sec., multiply by 2 - count for 60 sec. if irregular
respiration 16~20 per minute	- count for 15 sec., multiply by 4

blood pressure
diastolic: 60~ 90 mmHg
systolic: 95~140 mmHg
	- use appropriate size cuff
	  (pediatric cuff for children)
	- place 1 inch above antecubital fossa
	- apply not too loose
	
	- a difference of 5~10 mmHg between both
	  arms is normal

1.11.) <u>PREOPERATIVE CARE</u>

IMPLEMENTATION
- Solid food allowed 8-10 hours before surgery
- Clear fluids allowed 4 hours before surgery
- Assess client's understanding of procedure
- Provide time for client to express concerns
  SKIN SHAVING:
- May actually increase risk of infection
- If required do immediately prior to surgery
- Avoid any scratches or skin abrasions
- Always shave in direction of hair growth (not against)

1.12.) <u>POSTOPERATIVE CARE</u>

Early ambulation reduces postoperative complications!

IMPLEMENTATION
PACU:
- Maintain airways - position client on side with neck extended
- Monitor level of consciousness and reflexes
- Monitor until vital signs are stable for 30 minutes
- Monitor body temperature hourly
- Watch for paralytic ileus (absent bowel sounds)
  GENERAL:
- Turn client every 2 hours
- Deep breaths to prevent atelectasis (or incentive spirometry)
- Cough to remove chest secretions
  (place hands over abdominal incision site to act as a splint)
- Monitor drainage for color and amount

*Hearing returns more quickly than other senses: Avoid saying
anything that might distress client, even if she appears asleep!*

13

1.13.) WOUND CARE

PRIMARY INTENTION	SECONDARY INTENTION
• aseptic sharp wounds	• ulcers, traumatic injuries, infected wounds
• minimal tissue damage • minimal scar formation	• intentionally left open until granulation tissue forms or until aseptic
• (keloid may still form)	

> ➤ **Dry dressing:** for wounds closed by primary intention
> ➤ **Wet dressing:** for open and/or infected wounds
>   (debris and necrotic tissue are absorbed into gauze)
> ➤ **Occlusive dressing (petroleum gauze):** around chest tubes, fistulas
>   (to protect from air- or moisture-born infections)

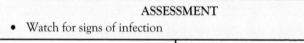

ASSESSMENT
- Watch for signs of infection

↓

IMPLEMENTATION
- Dressing protects wound from mechanical injury
- Pressure dressing if bleeding profusely
- Wet dressing with antimicrobial solution if prone to infection
- Monitor drainage: largest amount occurs in first 24 hours

As soon as wound is dry and clean the dressing should be removed to eliminate conditions for bacterial growth (warmth & moisture).

NUTRITION
&
CALCULATIONS

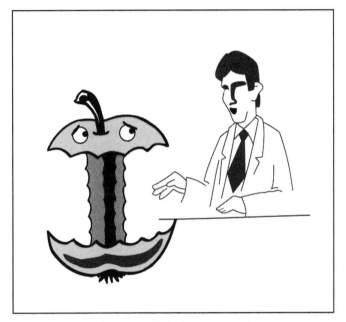

"Well, I am not totally sure, but you either have anorexia or bulimia."

Part A : NUTRITION

2.1.) HEALTH PROMOTION

Up to 35% of all cancer deaths may be preventable with a better diet!

	RECOMMENDATIONS
fat (1g=9kcal)	- no more than 30% of calories - avoid butter, lard and coconut oil
fiber	20 to 30g daily
fruit/vegetable	5 or 6 servings a day
meat	- prefer fish and white meat - remove skin and fat - avoid organ meats - avoid sausage and bacon
eggs	- avoid egg yolks

Example: In an average diet of 2,000 calories/day up to 600 kcal may come from fat. Each gram of fat contains 9 calories. Since 600/9=67, the average diet should contain not more than 67g of fat!

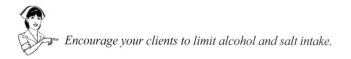

Encourage your clients to limit alcohol and salt intake.

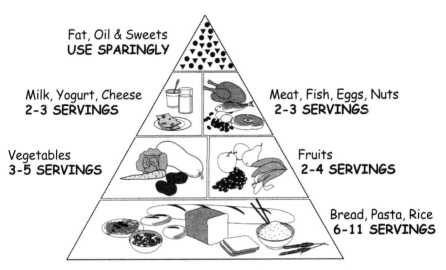

Fat, Oil & Sweets
USE SPARINGLY

Milk, Yogurt, Cheese
2-3 SERVINGS

Meat, Fish, Eggs, Nuts
2-3 SERVINGS

Vegetables
3-5 SERVINGS

Fruits
2-4 SERVINGS

Bread, Pasta, Rice
6-11 SERVINGS

SOURCE: U.S. Department of Agriculture/U.S. Department of Health and Human Services

SMOKING:

- ➢ 30% of all cancers are related to smoking!
- ➢ More than 50% of all smokers started before age of 16!

INCREASED RISK FOR:
- ➢ Lung cancer
- ➢ Cancer of the esophagus, colon, pancreas and bladder
- ➢ Chronic obstructive lung disease
- ➢ Coronary heart disease
- ➢ Peripheral vascular disease

EXERCISE:

- ➢ Helps to control weight
- ➢ Helps to control blood pressure
- ➢ Increases HDL (="good cholesterol")
- ➢ Lowers risk of coronary heart disease

- ➢ *Recommend walking, swimming, biking and low-impact aerobics.*

17

2.2.) LOW-PROTEIN DIET

indications	renal failure liver failure
purpose	to limit ammonium production
reduce	meat, eggs, milk products
encourage	carbohydrates (pasta, vegetable etc.) *supplement with essential amino acids*

2.3.) HIGH-PROTEIN DIET

indications	undernutrition burns nephrotic syndrome
purpose	to support protein synthesis
reduce	-
encourage	meat, fish, dairy products

 Extensive tissue repair may require up to 6,000 kcal/day !

2.4.) LOW-CHOLESTEROL DIET

indications	cardiovascular disease diabetes mellitus
purpose	to decrease risk of coronary heart disease
reduce	fried food! egg yolk shell fish liver, pork
encourage	broiled or steamed food! fruits, vegetables chicken meat vegetable oils

2.5.) LOW-FAT DIET

indications	malabsorption syndrome gallbladder diseases cystic fibrosis
purpose	to lower overall fat intake
reduce	fatty meat, gravy cream, chocolate nuts
encourage	vegetable, fruits lean meats fish

19

2.6.) DIABETIC DIET

indication	diabetes mellitus
purpose	to control plasma glucose levels
principles	Each meal should contain carbohydrates, fat and protein. Avoid skipping or delaying meals. Frequent, small meals may give better glucose control. Unplanned activity: add snack to avoid hypoglycemia.

Weight reduction is the primary treatment for NIDDM !

2.7.) BLAND DIET

indications	gastric and duodenal ulcers
purpose	to avoid irritation
reduce	hot spices, raw foods
encourage	milk, butter, eggs white bread, broiled potatoes

A bland diet used to be prescribed routinely for gastric or duodenal ulcers, but since the discovery that most peptic ulcer disease is caused by the bacterium *H. pylori* it is treated with antibiotics and a bland diet is rarely indicated. Instead, a well balanced diet with meals at regular intervals is recommended.

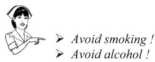

➢ *Avoid smoking !*
➢ *Avoid alcohol !*

2.8.) LOW-SODIUM DIET

indications	hypertension
	edema due to:
	- congestive heart failure
	- liver cirrhosis
	- nephrotic syndrome
	- preeclampsia
purpose	to decrease sodium/fluid load
reduce	canned food
	salted snacks
	smoked meat
	ham, bacon
	soy sauce
encourage	salt substitute: potassium chloride

21

2.9.) HIGH-POTASSIUM DIET

indications	thiazide diuretics diabetic ketoacidosis burns chronic vomiting
purpose	to avoid potassium depletion
encourage	bananas, prunes avocado soy beans

2.10.) OTHER DIETS

	INDICATIONS
high fiber diet	constipation diverticulitis may reduce risk of colon cancer!
low fiber diet	Crohn's disease diverticulitis (active inflammation)
low purine diet	uric acid stones gout
high acid ash (*cranberry juice, prunes, meat*)	calcium stones

2.11.) <u>VITAMINS</u>

	SOURCES	DEFICIENCY CAUSES
A	liver, egg yolk, carrots	poor night vision growth retardation (children)
D	milk, sunshine	bone deformities - children: rickets - adults: osteomalacia
E	vegetable oils	deficiency is very rare
K	liver, egg yolk, green leafy vegetables	bleeding disorders (deficiency of coagulation factors)
C	citrus fruits	scurvy (tooth loss, impaired wound healing)
B1	liver, meat	peripheral neuropathy Wernicke-Korsakoff *(alcoholics!)*
B2	liver, meat	inflammation of tongue and lips (glossitis and cheilosis)
B12	liver, meat	anemia neuropathy
olic acid	green leafy vegetable	anemia

Vitamin deficiency (especially B group) is common in alcoholics!
Folic acid deficiency is common in pregnant women!

Part B : CALCULATIONS

1 mL = 1 cc, 1 gtt = 1 drop

2.12.) DOSAGE CALCULATIONS

$$D/H \cdot Q = x$$

D: desired dose (from doctor's order)
H: dose on **hand** (from drug label)
Q: quantity that contains the dose you have on hand

EXAMPLE:

Doctor's order: 90 mg p.o.
Drug label: 1 tablet contains 60 mg

D = 90 mg,   **H** = 60 mg,   **Q** = 1 tablet

(90 / 60) · 1 = 1.5 → you should give 1.5 tablets

EXAMPLE:

Doctor's order: 7,000 U s.c.
Drug label: 5,000 U per 10 mL

D = 7,000 U   **H** = 5,000 U,   **Q** = 10 mL

(7,000 / 5,000) · 10 = 14 → you should give 14 mL

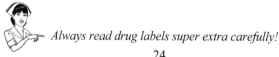

Always read drug labels super extra carefully!
24

2.13.) <u>IV CALCULATIONS</u>

% = grams per 100 mL solution

<u>EXAMPLE:</u>

D5W (5% dextrose in water) contains 5 g / 100 mL = 50 g dextrose / L
Normal saline (0.9% NaCl) contains 0.9 g / 100 mL = 9 g NaCl / L

V/T · drop factor = gtt/min

V: volume to infuse <u>in mL</u>
T: time for infusion <u>in minutes</u>
drop factor: number of drops per mL (depends on tubing used!)

<u>EXAMPLE:</u>

Doctor's order: infuse 200 mL / hour
Drop set: 10 gtt/mL

V = 200 mL,   T = 60 min,   **drop factor** = 10 gtt/mL

(200 / 60) · 10 = 33.3 → you should infuse at a rate of 33 gtt/min

<u>EXAMPLE:</u>

Doctor's order: infuse 1 L D5W in 6 hours
Drop set: 10 gtt/mL

V = 1,000 mL,   T = 360 min,   **drop factor** = 10 gtt/mL

(1,000 / 360) · 10 = 27.8 → you should infuse at a rate of 28 gtt/min

FLUIDS
&
ELECTROLYTES

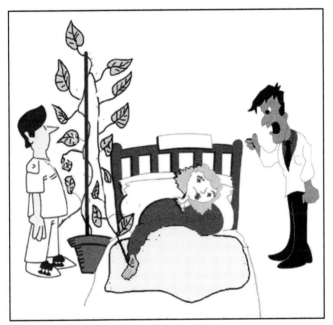

I said *"Put in an IV"* what could be simpler?

3.1.) <u>DIFFUSION & OSMOSIS</u>

➤ **Solvent:** the medium (usually water) that contains some particles.
➤ **Solutes:** particles that are dissolved in solvent: salts, sugars, amino acids...

DIFFUSION

Particles move from an area of high concentration to an area of low concentration until equilibrium is reached:

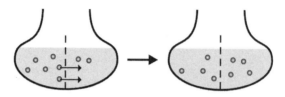

Examples:

☞ Oxygen moves from an area of high concentration (alveoli) to an area of low concentration (lung capillaries).

☞ CO_2 moves from an area of high concentration (lung capillaries) to an area of low concentration (alveoli).

☞ Interstitial lung diseases thicken the alveolar walls and reduce permeability (diffusion barrier) → impaired gas exchange.

OSMOSIS

If a diffusion barrier prevents the particles from reaching osmotic equilibrium, water will move to the side of higher osmotic concentration until equilibrium is reached:

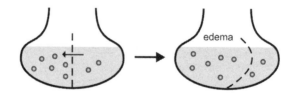

edema

Example:

☞ If albumin (blood protein) is lost, the osmolarity of plasma becomes less than that of the extracellular fluid. As a result, water moves from the capillaries to the extracellular space and forms edema.

3.2.) ACID / BASE PHYSIOLOGY

Our metabolism constantly produces acids (H⁺). If these were not buffered the plasma would become so acidic that life were impossible.

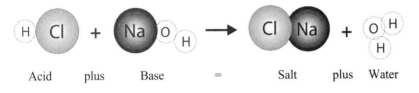

| Acid | plus | Base | = | Salt | plus | Water |

➢ **Strong acids dissociate completely:**

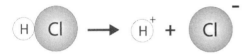

➢ **Weak acids dissociate partially.**
➢ **Buffer = weak acid + its salt** (for example H_2CO_3 + $NaHCO_3$)
  When dissolved in water they form an equilibrium:

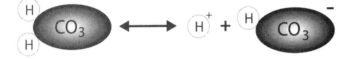

Add acid (H⁺): equilibrium shifts to the left: **H_2CO_3 ← HCO_3^-**

Remove acid (H⁺): equilibrium shifts to the right: H_2CO_3 → **HCO_3^-**

Our body has 2 additional defense mechanisms against too much acid:

1. If too much H_2CO_3 is produced by the above reactions, the lungs can remove it in the form of CO_2.

   ☞ Inability to remove CO_2 due to hypoventilation causes acidosis.

   ☞ Removal of too much CO_2 by hyperventilation causes alkalosis.

2. The kidneys can recover buffer base HCO_3^- as needed to compensate for acidosis.

   ☞ Inability of the kidneys to recover HCO_3^- causes acidosis.

3.3.) ACID / BASE DISORDERS

A) HOW TO DRAW ARTERIAL BLOOD GASES:

- Draw into heparinized syringe
- Must be sterile
- Discard if in contact with room air
- Keep on ice, transport to lab immediately
- Apply pressure to puncture site for 5~10 minutes

B) HOW TO ASSESS ARTERIAL BLOOD GASES:

- **First Step: check pH**
  pH < 7.35 (acidosis)
  pH = 7.4   (normal)
  pH > 7.45 (alkalosis)

- **Second Step: determine primary cause of disturbance**

  In case of acidosis: - if CO_2 > 40 mmHg: cause is respiratory
  - if HCO_3^- < 24 mmHg: cause is metabolic

  In case of alkalosis: - if CO_2 < 40 mmHg: cause is respiratory
  - if HCO_3^- > 24 mmHg: cause is metabolic

A normal pH may indicate perfectly normal condition, or it may indicate a compensated imbalance. For example, a client with metabolic acidosis initially has low pH and low plasma bicarbonate. The client starts to hyperventilate (lowers CO_2) until the pH normalizes.

C) CAUSES OF ACID / BASE DISORDERS:

	blood pH	primary disturbance	clinical causes
simple hypoxia	normal	normal	- acute respiratory distress - pneumonia
respiratory acidosis	< 7.35	CO_2 ↑	**hypoventilation:** - COPD - lung edema - brainstem injury
metabolic acidosis	< 7.35	HCO_3^- ↓	- diabetes (ketoacidosis) - shock (lactate) - diarrhea [1]
respiratory alkalosis	> 7.45	CO_2 ↓	**hyperventilation:** - high altitude - anxiety
metabolic alkalosis	> 7.45	HCO_3^- ↑	- vomiting [2] - diuretics

[1] *loss of bicarbonate*
[2] *loss of acid*

3.4.) <u>RESPIRATORY ACIDOSIS</u>

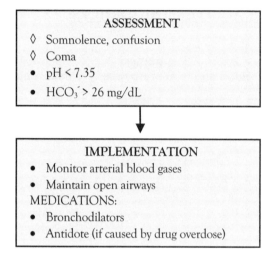

ASSESSMENT
◊ Somnolence, confusion
◊ Coma
• pH < 7.35
• $HCO_3^- > 26$ mg/dL

IMPLEMENTATION
• Monitor arterial blood gases
• Maintain open airways
MEDICATIONS:
• Bronchodilators
• Antidote (if caused by drug overdose)

3.5.) <u>METABOLIC ACIDOSIS</u>

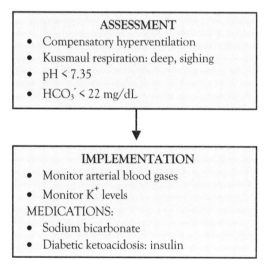

ASSESSMENT
• Compensatory hyperventilation
• Kussmaul respiration: deep, sighing
• pH < 7.35
• $HCO_3^- < 22$ mg/dL

IMPLEMENTATION
• Monitor arterial blood gases
• Monitor K^+ levels
MEDICATIONS:
• Sodium bicarbonate
• Diabetic ketoacidosis: insulin

3.6.) <u>RESPIRATORY ALKALOSIS</u>

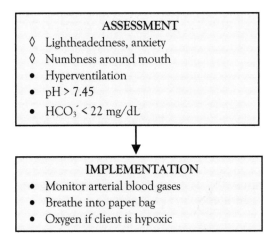

ASSESSMENT
◊ Lightheadedness, anxiety
◊ Numbness around mouth
• Hyperventilation
• pH > 7.45
• HCO_3^- < 22 mg/dL

IMPLEMENTATION
• Monitor arterial blood gases
• Breathe into paper bag
• Oxygen if client is hypoxic

Anxiety → hyperventilation → respiratory alkalosis → more anxiety...

3.7.) <u>METABOLIC ALKALOSIS</u>

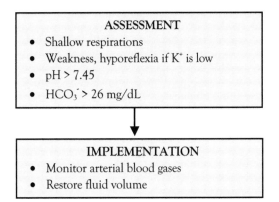

ASSESSMENT
• Shallow respirations
• Weakness, hyporeflexia if K^+ is low
• pH > 7.45
• HCO_3^- > 26 mg/dL

IMPLEMENTATION
• Monitor arterial blood gases
• Restore fluid volume

3.8.) SODIUM LEVELS

➤ Na^+ levels usually reflect the body's water content, rather than body's Na^+ content, for example, high Na^+ levels are usually due to loss of water!

CAUSES:

hypernatremia **client dehydrated**	**- indicates water loss** - diarrhea, sweating, renal losses
hypernatremia **client overhydrated**	**- indicates net Na^+ gain** - Cushing's syndrome - hyperaldosteronism
hyponatremia low osmolarity	**- indicates water retention** - renal failure - excessive ADH production
hyponatremia normal or high osmolarity	**- sodium replaced by other solutes** - hyperlipidemia - hyperglycemia (diabetes mellitus) - hyperproteinemia (multiple myeloma)

3.9.) <u>SIMPLE DEHYDRATION</u>
Water and electrolytes are lost in the same proportion

```
ASSESSMENT
```
- Poor skin turgor
- Sunken eyes
- Dry mucous membranes
- Dark urine, increased specific gravity
- Increased hematocrit

↓

```
IMPLEMENTATION
```
- Fluid replacement
- Weigh client daily
- Monitor intake and output
- Monitor urine specific gravity

3.10.) <u>OVERHYDRATION</u>

```
ASSESSMENT
```
- Increased blood pressure
- Increased central venous pressure
- Distended neck veins
- Pitting edema
- Pulmonary edema → crackles

↓

```
IMPLEMENTATION
```
- Semi-Fowler's position
- Fluid restriction
- Weigh client daily
- Low-sodium diet
- Diuretics as ordered

3.11.) POTASSIUM LEVELS

> ➤ K⁺ is the major cation of the <u>intracellular</u> fluid.
> ➤ Small changes in extracellular K⁺ concentration are very significant!

CAUSES:

hypokalemia	**- hyperaldosteronism (Conn syndrome)** *excessive production of mineralocorticoids by adrenal glands* **- potassium loss** - renal loss: diuretics - gastrointestinal loss: diarrhea laxative abuse (common!) **- transcellular shift** - alkalosis - acute glucose load - insulin excess
hyperkalemia	**- hypoaldosteronism (Addison's disease)** *lack of mineralocorticoid production by adrenal glands* **- artifact:** RBC hemolysis during blood drawing **- transcellular shift** - acidosis

Vigorous drawing of blood may destroy red blood cells and result in artificially elevated K⁺ levels.

3.12.) <u>HYPERKALEMIA</u>

ASSESSMENT
◊ Irritability
- Diarrhea
- Cardiac arrhythmias
- Cardiac arrest

↓

IMPLEMENTATION
- Monitor ECG
- Insulin plus IV glucose to redistribute K^+
- Fluids to increase urinary output

High K^+ solutions are used during cardiac surgery to temporarily arrest the heart beat.

3.13.) <u>HYPOKALEMIA</u>

ASSESSMENT
- Muscle weakness and cramps
- Constipation

↓

IMPLEMENTATION
- Monitor ECG, especially if client is on digitalis!
- Carefully replace potassium
- *Never give IV bolus of potassium!*

Chronic use of laxatives often results in K^+ loss, which then worsens the constipation !

3.14.) CALCIUM LEVELS

➤ Ca^{2+} plays a crucial role in all "excitable tissues" (heart, muscles, nerves)
➤ Small changes in extracellular Ca^{2+} concentration are very significant!

CAUSES:

hypocalcemia	**- chronic renal failure** (high phosphate, low calcium levels) - hypoparathyroidism - lack of dietary Ca^{2+} and vit. D
hypercalcemia	**- cancer metastases to bones** - hyperparathyroidism - vitamin D poisoning

---

> *Free (=effective) Ca^{2+} depends on pH:*
> ➤ *Acidosis* → *high free Ca^{2+}*
> ➤ *Alkalosis* → *low free Ca^{2+}*

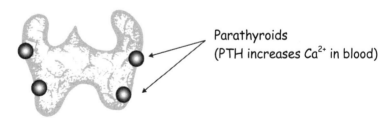

Parathyroids
(PTH increases Ca^{2+} in blood)

3.15.) HYPERCALCEMIA

ASSESSMENT
◊ Anorexia, nausea
◊ Abdominal pain

↓

IMPLEMENTATION
• Carefully increase client mobility
• Avoid trauma: risk of pathological fractures!
• Avoid large doses of vitamin D

3.16.) HYPOCALCEMIA

ASSESSMENT
◊ Tingling
◊ Numbness
• Hyperactive reflexes, tetany
• Chvostek sign, Trousseau sign

↓

IMPLEMENTATION
• Promote regular milk intake
• Keep 10% Ca-gluconate on hand

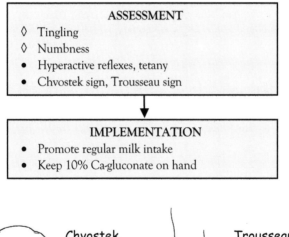

Chvostek Sign

Trousseau Sign

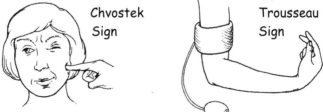

From *The Lippincott Manual of Nursing Practice*, 6th edition, p. 713, edited by S.M. Nettina.
Copyright 1996 by Lippincott-Raven Publishers, Philadelphia, PA. Used with permission.

3.17.) IV SOLUTIONS

➤ **Osmolarity:** total concentration of osmotically active solutes in a fluid
➤ **Isotonic solution:** solution with same osmolarity as human plasma
➤ **Hypertonic solution:** makes blood cells shrink
➤ **Hypotonic solution:** makes blood cells expand

	TONICITY	COMPOSITION
5% DW	isotonic	235 mOsm/L dextrose *(170 kcal/L)*
10% DW	hypertonic	561 mOsm/L dextrose *(340 kcal/L)*
0.9 % NS	isotonic	154 mM/L Na⁺ 154 mM/L Cl⁻
lactate Ringer	isotonic	148 mM/L Na⁺ 4 mM/L K⁺ 4.5 mM/L Ca²⁺ 156 mM/L Cl⁻

DW = dextrose in water, NS = normal saline

5% DW is initially isotonic when infused intravenously. As the glucose diffuses into the cells and is metabolized however, the net effect will be infusion of a hypotonic solution !

On the other hand 0.9% NS remains isotonic because there is no net movement of osmotically active molecules.

CARDIOVASCULAR
DISEASES

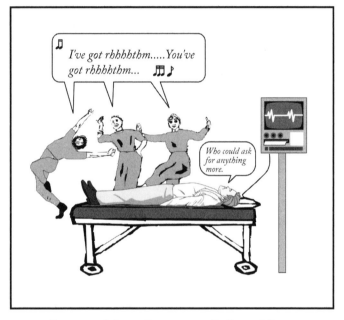

Successful cardiac resuscitation at the
George Gershwin Memorial Hospital

4.1.) PHYSIOLOGY

Cardiac output = stroke volume · heart rate

Note that at very high heart rates the cardiac output decreases because of a decrease i stroke volume (less time for the ventricles to fill during diastole).

Blood pressure = cardiac output · vascular resistance

High blood pressure can be due to increased cardiac output or increased resistance to blood flow from vasoconstriction.

Systolic blood pressure: is an indicator of cardiac output
Diastolic blood pressure: is an indicator of vascular resistance to blood flow

	ACTION
sinus node	- pacemaker of heart - P waves on ECG
AV node	- passes electrical excitation from atria to ventricles with some delay - PR interval on ECG
vagus nerve	- slows heart rate *(sinus node)* - slows conduction from atria to ventricles *(AV node)*
sympathetic nerves	- increase heart rate - increase force of contraction *(muscles of atria and ventricles)*

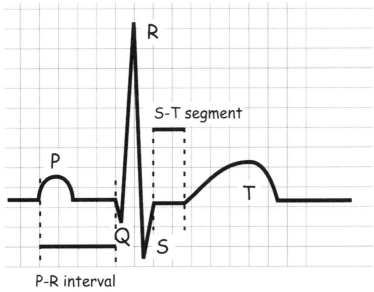

P-R interval
0.12 ~ 0.20 sec

4.2.) SIGNS & SYMPTOMS

orthopnea difficulty breathing in supine position	- left heart failure (congested lung blood vessels)
pulsus alternans beat to beat change in pulse amplitude	- left heart failure
pulsus paradoxus exaggerated decline of pulse pressure during inspiration	- cardiac tamponade - constrictive pericarditis - massive pulmonary embolism
Kussmaul's sign distention of jugular veins with inspiration	- constrictive pericarditis

4.3.) <u>HYPERTENSION</u>

```
┌─────────────────────────────────────────────────────────────┐
│                         ASSESSMENT                          │
│  ◊  Asymptomatic (="the silent killer")                     │
│  ◊  Headache, blurred vision only if greatly elevated BP    │
│  •  BP > 140/90 mmHg                                         │
│  •  Assess possible damage to kidneys                       │
└─────────────────────────────────────────────────────────────┘
```

```
┌─────────────────────────────────────────────────────────────┐
│                      IMPLEMENTATION                         │
│  DIET:                                                       │
│  •  Reduce weight!                                           │
│  •  Reduce salt intake to < 2g/day                          │
│  •  Reduce cholesterol and saturated fats                   │
│  MEDICATIONS:                                               │
│  •  Diuretics, β-blockers                                   │
└─────────────────────────────────────────────────────────────┘
```

```
┌─────────────────────────────────────────────────────────────┐
│                     CLIENT EDUCATION                        │
│  •  Promote diet and lifestyle changes                      │
│  •  Teach importance of compliance with medications         │
└─────────────────────────────────────────────────────────────┘
```

```
┌─────────────────────────────────────────────────────────────┐
│                         EVALUATION                          │
│  •  Evaluate other risk factors of coronary heart disease   │
└─────────────────────────────────────────────────────────────┘
```

In most cases of hypertension <u>no medical cause</u> can be found (this is called "essential hypertension"). Before a diagnosis of "essential hypertension" is made other causes should be excluded:

- Renal diseases
- Renovascular diseases
- Cushing's syndrome (elevated cortisol levels)
- Aldosteronism (elevated mineralocorticoid levels)

44

4.4.) <u>CORONARY HEART DISEASE</u>

Heart disease causes 1/4 of all deaths in the US

Risk Factors:

FIXED	MODIFIABLE
- male sex - family history - older age	- cigarette smoking - high LDL - low HDL - diabetes mellitus - hypertension

LDL = "bad cholesterol", HDL = "good cholesterol"

cholesterol	**TC = HDL + LDL + triglycerides/5** TC > 240 mg/dL = increased risk for CHD LDL > 160 mg/dL = increased risk for CHD HDL/LDL > 0.4 desirable
triglycerides	- increased levels with age - TG > 200 mg/dL = increased risk for CHD - estrogen and oral contraceptives increase triglycerides

TC = total cholesterol,   CHD = coronary heart disease

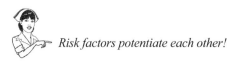 *Risk factors potentiate each other!*

4.5.) CHEST PAIN

classic angina	◊ substernal pain ◊ transient (<10 min) ◊ provoked by exercise • relieved by rest or nitrates
unstable angina	◊ change in pattern (more frequent, severe or prolonged) ◊ angina at rest or at night
variant angina (=Prinzmetal angina)	◊ due to coronary artery vasospasm ◊ not provoked by exercise!
myocardial infarction	◊ substernal pain → arm, shoulder, jaw ◊ lasts > 30 min • not relieved by rest or nitrates • **Elevated enzymes:** cardiac troponin CTnT creatine kinase CK lactate dehydrogenase LDH

CORONARY ARTERIES:

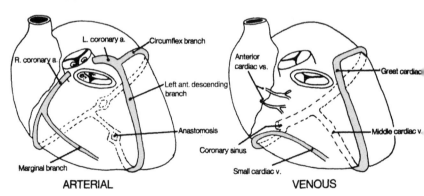

ARTERIAL   VENOUS

From Goldberg: *Clinical Anatomy Made Ridiculously Simple*, MedMaster, 2007

46

4.6.) OTHER CAUSES OF CHEST PAIN

 These may sometimes be confused with myocardial infarction!

	KEY FEATURES
pulmonary embolism	- sudden onset dyspnea / tachypnea - pleuritic chest pain - vomiting blood indicates pulmonary infarction
pneumothorax	- sudden onset sharp pain - aggravated by breathing - **hyperresonant** to percussion
pleurisy	- well localized pain - aggravated by breathing - **dull** to percussion
peptic ulcer	- burning, gnawing pain - lower substernal area, epigastrium - often relieved by food or antacids
psychosomatic	- sharp, often localized to a point - usually of short duration

4.7.) <u>ANGINA PECTORIS</u>

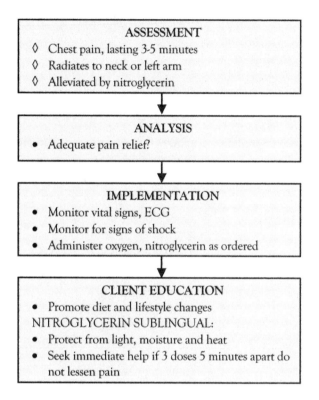

ASSESSMENT
- ◊ Chest pain, lasting 3-5 minutes
- ◊ Radiates to neck or left arm
- ◊ Alleviated by nitroglycerin

ANALYSIS
- Adequate pain relief?

IMPLEMENTATION
- Monitor vital signs, ECG
- Monitor for signs of shock
- Administer oxygen, nitroglycerin as ordered

CLIENT EDUCATION
- Promote diet and lifestyle changes
NITROGLYCERIN SUBLINGUAL:
- Protect from light, moisture and heat
- Seek immediate help if 3 doses 5 minutes apart do not lessen pain

Unstable angina: *- lasts longer than 15 minutes*
- increases in intensity
- occurs at rest

<u>Teach client importance of reducing risk factors</u>:
1. Stop smoking
2. Control blood pressure
3. Lower lipids aggressively
4. Control blood glucose in diabetic patients

4.8.) MYOCARDIAL INFARCTION

ASSESSMENT
◊ Crushing substernal pain
◊ lasts > 30 minutes
◊ not relieved by rest or nitroglycerin
- ECG changes: ST changes, Q waves (transmural infarction)
- Cardiac enzymes: CTnT detectable 6-12 hours after MI
  more specific than the other enzymes

ANALYSIS
- Adequate cardiac output?
- Adequate pain relief?
- Coping with anxiety?

IMPLEMENTATION
- Bed rest for 24-48 hours (semi-Fowler's position)
- Avoid straining, since this increases blood pressure
  (stool softeners if needed)
- Monitor ECG, ABGs and blood pressure
- Monitor for complications: congestive heart failure, arrhythmias
MEDICATIONS:
- Morphine: give IV (avoid IM injections in cardiac patients!)
- Oxygen
- Heparin anticoagulation

CLIENT EDUCATION
- Slowly increase physical activity
- Promote dietary and lifestyle changes

Frothy, pink tinged sputum indicates pulmonary edema:
Report immediately !

4.9.) COMPLICATIONS OF MI

Monitor every post-MI patient very carefully for these complications:

EARLY:

arrhythmia	◊ dizziness, palpitations • syncope
congestive heart failure	◊ dyspnea, orthopnea • rales, wheezes (cardiac asthma) • cardiogenic shock
pericarditis	**occurs 1~3 days after MI** ◊ pleuritic pain, non-responsive to nitrates ◊ self-limited

DAYS TO WEEKS:

myocardial rupture	• tamponade, shock, death • typically occurs with **small infarcts** !
papillary muscle rupture	• hyperacute onset pulmonary edema • loud systolic murmur (mitral regurgitation)

WEEKS TO MONTHS:

ventricular aneurysm	• reduced cardiac output • mural thrombi → arterial emboli

4.10.) ARRHYTHMIAS

sick sinus node	- sudden tachycardias / bradycardias - normal P waves on ECG
AV block – 1ˢᵗ degree	- PR interval prolonged (> 0.2 s) - every P followed by a QRS
AV block – 2ⁿᵈ degree	- occasional QRS dropouts
AV block – 3ʳᵈ degree (complete)	- QRS independent of P waves (ventricles beat independently from atria)

> ➢ Ventricular flutter is immediately life-threatening!
> ➢ Atrial flutter is much less serious.

4.11.) PACEMAKERS

POSTOPERATIVE
- Continuous monitoring of ECG
- Monitor for signs of hemothorax (hypotension, restlessness)
- Monitor for signs of pneumothorax (dyspnea, absent breath sounds)
- Monitor for lead migration → tamponade (distended neck veins)
- Avoid underarm lifts when transferring patient

CLIENT EDUCATION
- Avoid heavy lifting
- Avoid difficult arm maneuvers, stretching or bending
- Report hiccups, palpitation or dizziness immediately
- *Caution with electromagnetic devices: Transformers, cautery, electric razors, anti-theft devices.*
- Carry ID card

4.12.) <u>CONGESTIVE HEART FAILURE</u>

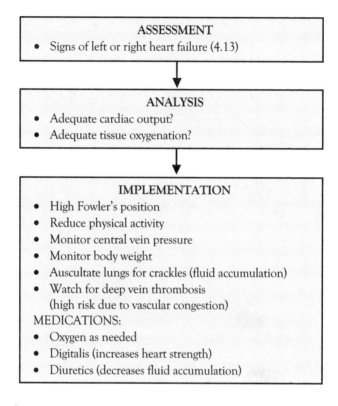

ASSESSMENT
- Signs of left or right heart failure (4.13)

ANALYSIS
- Adequate cardiac output?
- Adequate tissue oxygenation?

IMPLEMENTATION
- High Fowler's position
- Reduce physical activity
- Monitor central vein pressure
- Monitor body weight
- Auscultate lungs for crackles (fluid accumulation)
- Watch for deep vein thrombosis
  (high risk due to vascular congestion)

MEDICATIONS:
- Oxygen as needed
- Digitalis (increases heart strength)
- Diuretics (decreases fluid accumulation)

Watch for digitalis toxicity: *nausea, yellow color vision, arrhythmia.*
Watch for signs of hypokalemia: *weakness and muscle cramps.*

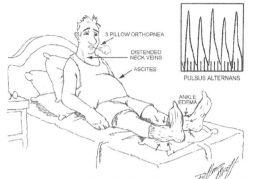

Modified from Chizner: *Clinical Cardiology Made Ridiculously Simple*, MedMaster, 2010

CLIENT EDUCATION

DIET:
- Restrict salt and fluid
- Avoid food high in sodium
- Avoid potassium loss
  (unless potassium sparing diuretics are used)

4.13.) ASSESSMENT: HEART FAILURE

LEFT HEART FAILURE	RIGHT HEART FAILURE
SIGNS & SYMPTOMS:	
◊ dyspnea ◊ orthopnea ◊ non-productive cough at night • pulsus alternans	◊ pitting edema (ankles) ◊ weight gain ◊ nocturia • jugular vein distention • hepatomegaly
CAUSES:	
- ischemic heart disease - arterial hypertension - valvular disease	- left sided heart failure - lung disease - pulmonary hypertension
CONSEQUENCES:	
pulmonary congestion: - dyspnea, orthopnea renal hypoperfusion: - salt retention	increased venous pressure: - edema - liver congestion, ascites

4.14.) ASSESSMENT: SHOCK

Flow of blood to peripheral tissues inadequate to sustain life.

SHOCK TYPE	SIGNS AND CAUSES
heart failure (cardiogenic shock)	• **cool, pale skin** • **distended neck veins** - myocardial infarction - cardiomyopathy - arrhythmias
blood loss (hypovolemic shock)	• **cool, pale skin** • **collapsed neck veins** - hemorrhage - Addison's crisis
sepsis (septic shock)	• **warm, dry skin** • **edema despite hypovolemia** - gram negative bacteria (endotoxins)
anaphylaxis (allergic shock)	• **pruritus, urticaria** • **respiratory distress** - immune reaction (type IV mediated by IgE antibodies)

4.15.) HYPOVOLEMIC SHOCK

CAUSES:
➢ Hemorrhage (internal or external bleeding)
➢ Fluid loss from wounds (especially in burn patients!)
➢ Neurogenic → Vasodilation → reduced cardiac filling

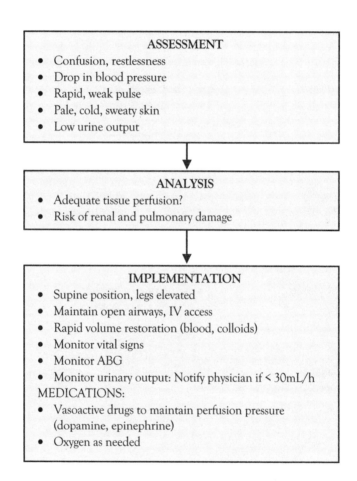

ASSESSMENT
- Confusion, restlessness
- Drop in blood pressure
- Rapid, weak pulse
- Pale, cold, sweaty skin
- Low urine output

ANALYSIS
- Adequate tissue perfusion?
- Risk of renal and pulmonary damage

IMPLEMENTATION
- Supine position, legs elevated
- Maintain open airways, IV access
- Rapid volume restoration (blood, colloids)
- Monitor vital signs
- Monitor ABG
- Monitor urinary output: Notify physician if < 30mL/h
MEDICATIONS:
- Vasoactive drugs to maintain perfusion pressure (dopamine, epinephrine)
- Oxygen as needed

4.16.) PERICARDITIS

infectious	- **often preceded by "cold"** - viruses - tuberculosis - AIDS
metabolic	- **uremia** (kidney failure) - **myxedema** (hypothyroid)
post MI	- **early** (1-3 days after MI) self-limited, common

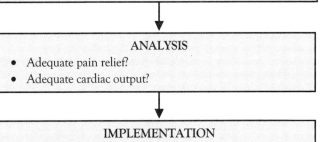

ASSESSMENT
◊ Mild or sharp pain over sternum
• Pericardial friction rub on auscultation
• Increased venous pressure → constrictive pericarditis

ANALYSIS
• Adequate pain relief?
• Adequate cardiac output?

IMPLEMENTATION
• Leaning forward may alleviate pain
• Monitor vital signs
• Check for signs of cardiac tamponade
MEDICATIONS:
• Salicylates, corticosteroids
• Antibiotics

4.17.) CARDIAC TAMPONADE
Accumulation of fluid in pericardial space

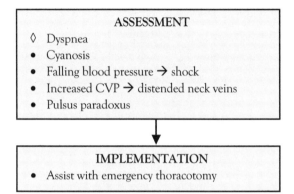

ASSESSMENT
◊ Dyspnea
• Cyanosis
• Falling blood pressure → shock
• Increased CVP → distended neck veins
• Pulsus paradoxus

IMPLEMENTATION
• Assist with emergency thoracotomy

4.18.) MYOCARDITIS

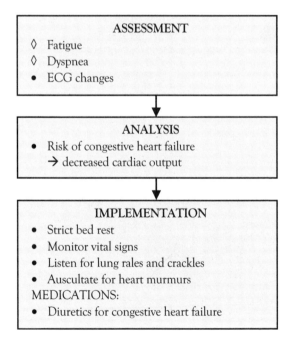

ASSESSMENT
◊ Fatigue
◊ Dyspnea
• ECG changes

ANALYSIS
• Risk of congestive heart failure
  → decreased cardiac output

IMPLEMENTATION
• Strict bed rest
• Monitor vital signs
• Listen for lung rales and crackles
• Auscultate for heart murmurs
MEDICATIONS:
• Diuretics for congestive heart failure

4.19.) RHEUMATIC HEART DISEASE

ACUTE RHEUMATIC FEVER	RHEUMATIC HEART DISEASE
occurs 1~4 weeks after tonsillitis (streptococcal infection)	- occurs many years after rheumatic fever - involves: mitral valve > aortic valve
affects children 5~15 years	manifests itself in adults
polyarthritis **carditis** - pericarditis - myocarditis - endocarditis **erythema** **subcutaneous nodules**	◊ **early: often asymptomatic** • **late: congestive heart failure**

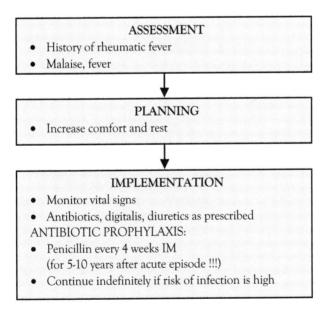

ASSESSMENT
- History of rheumatic fever
- Malaise, fever

PLANNING
- Increase comfort and rest

IMPLEMENTATION
- Monitor vital signs
- Antibiotics, digitalis, diuretics as prescribed
ANTIBIOTIC PROPHYLAXIS:
- Penicillin every 4 weeks IM
  (for 5-10 years after acute episode !!!)
- Continue indefinitely if risk of infection is high

4.20.) HEART VALVES

mitral stenosis	*increased left atrial and pulmonary pressure* ◊ dyspnea, orthopnea • atrial fibrillation
mitral regurgitation	*increased left atrial and ventricular work load* • pulmonary congestion
mitral valve prolapse	◊ palpitations ◊ atypical chest pain ◊ usually benign
aortic stenosis	*increased left ventricular work load* ◊ angina • fainting during exercise
aortic regurgitation	*increased left ventricular work load* • large pulse amplitude ("waterhammer pulse") **"FAMOUS SIGNS":** • **DeMusset:** head bobbing • **Traube:** pistol shot sounds heard over arteries • **Quincke:** pulsatile blushing of nail beds

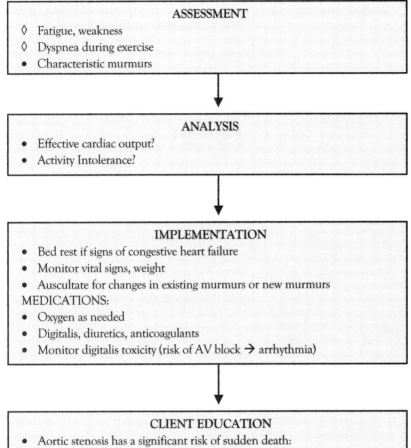

ASSESSMENT

◊ Fatigue, weakness
◊ Dyspnea during exercise
• Characteristic murmurs

ANALYSIS

• Effective cardiac output?
• Activity Intolerance?

IMPLEMENTATION

• Bed rest if signs of congestive heart failure
• Monitor vital signs, weight
• Auscultate for changes in existing murmurs or new murmurs
MEDICATIONS:
• Oxygen as needed
• Digitalis, diuretics, anticoagulants
• Monitor digitalis toxicity (risk of AV block → arrhythmia)

CLIENT EDUCATION

• Aortic stenosis has a significant risk of sudden death:
  Avoid strenuous exercise!
• All clients with aortic or mitral valve disease should receive prophylaxis
  against endocarditis (see 4.20)

4.21.) CARDIOMYOPATHY

dilated (congestive)	**- dilated ventricle, normal wall thickness** **- left and right ventricular failure** - alcohol - viral infections
hypertrophic	**- ventricular hypertrophy** **- small cavity** **- septum may obstruct outflow** - often genetic
restrictive	**- ventricular stiffness** **(restricts diastolic filling)** - amyloidosis - sarcoidosis - hemochromatosis

Hypertrophic cardiomyopathy: If client develops chest pain, provide bed rest and elevate feet to improve venous return. Nitroglycerin could worsen chest pain in these clients !

NORMAL   DILATED

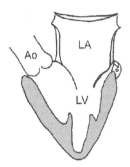   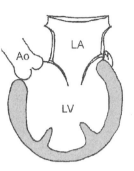

In the normal heart, the left intraventricular chamber is cone shaped, tapering at the apex. In dilated (congestive) cardiomyopathy, the LV chamber becomes dilated and nearly spherical in diastole.

HYPERTROPHIC   RESTRICTIVE

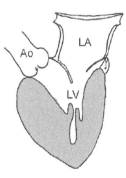   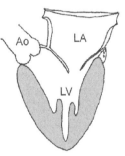

In hypertrophic cardiomyopathy, the LV cavity is very small in diastole, often asymmetric. In restrictive cardiomyopathy, the myocardium is very stiff and the LV cavity smaller than normal.

Modified from Chizner: *Clinical Cardiology Made Ridiculously Simple*, MedMaster, 2010

4.22.) <u>ENDOCARDITIS</u>

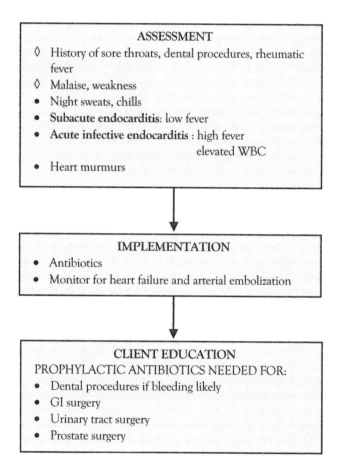

ASSESSMENT
◊ History of sore throats, dental procedures, rheumatic fever
◊ Malaise, weakness
• Night sweats, chills
• **Subacute endocarditis:** low fever
• **Acute infective endocarditis :** high fever
                                    elevated WBC
• Heart murmurs

IMPLEMENTATION
• Antibiotics
• Monitor for heart failure and arterial embolization

CLIENT EDUCATION
PROPHYLACTIC ANTIBIOTICS NEEDED FOR:
• Dental procedures if bleeding likely
• GI surgery
• Urinary tract surgery
• Prostate surgery

4.23.) BLOOD VESSELS

arteriosclerosis	*- calcification and narrowing of blood vessels* *- affects large and medium vessels* • claudication: insufficient blood supply to leg muscles → pain in calf when walking, quickly relieved by rest
arterial embolism	*atrial fibrillation → risk of thromboembolia* ◊ sudden onset ◊ painful • absent pulse
Raynaud's phenomenon	• vasospasm of finger arteries • cyanosis followed by hyperemia *(white → blue → red)* • precipitated by cold or emotional upset **causes:** - cold antibodies - connective tissue diseases - neurologic disorders
thrombophlebitis (inflammation of veins)	◊ usually painful
phlebothrombosis (thrombus formation)	◊ often asymptomatic !!! ◊ high risk of lung embolism

 Early postoperative ambulation reduces risk of phlebothrombosis !

4.24.) <u>ARTERIOSCLEROSIS</u>

Loss of elasticity and thickening of vessel wall → narrow lumen

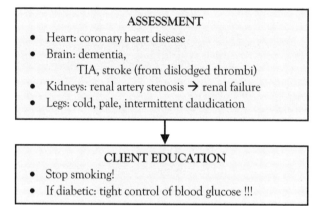

ASSESSMENT
- Heart: coronary heart disease
- Brain: dementia,
      TIA, stroke (from dislodged thrombi)
- Kidneys: renal artery stenosis → renal failure
- Legs: cold, pale, intermittent claudication

CLIENT EDUCATION
- Stop smoking!
- If diabetic: tight control of blood glucose !!!

4.25.) <u>RAYNAUD'S DISEASE</u>
Vasospasm of arteries in hand

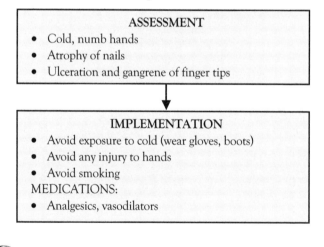

ASSESSMENT
- Cold, numb hands
- Atrophy of nails
- Ulceration and gangrene of finger tips

IMPLEMENTATION
- Avoid exposure to cold (wear gloves, boots)
- Avoid any injury to hands
- Avoid smoking
MEDICATIONS:
- Analgesics, vasodilators

Placing hands in warm water may terminate acute attack !

4.26.) <u>ANEURYSMS</u>

Weakened arterial wall → local distention → risk of rupture

	KEY FEATURES
atherosclerotic	- mainly abdominal aorta - a/w hypertension
syphilitic	- mainly ascending aorta - positive lab test for syphilis (VDRL)
dissecting	- aorta (ascending or descending) - a/w hypertension
berry	- intracranial arteries - congenital

ASSESSMENT
◊ Often asymptomatic
- Abdominal aneurysm: Pulsating mass
- Dissecting aneurysm: Sudden tearing pain

↓

IMPLEMENTATION
- Monitor vital signs
- Monitor for signs of shock
- Type and cross-match blood

Surgical removal of aortic aneurysm is indicated if diameter > 5 cm.
(very high risk of rupture and sudden death!)

4.27.) VASCULITIS

Inflammation of blood vessels – usually due to autoimmune process

Henoch Schönlein	**affects small vessels of skin, joints** (also GI tract and kidneys) ◊ abdominal pain • arthritis • skin rash (feet, legs, buttock) - purpura
polyarteritis nodosa	**affects small and medium vessels of many organs (kidneys, heart and GI tract)** ◊ abdominal pain ◊ weakness • fever Often "nonspecific" → difficult to diagnose
giant cell arteritis	**inflammation of temporal artery** ◊ malaise • fever • muscle and joint aches • red, tender, swollen temporal artery *Risk of blindness if not treated immediately!!!*

4.28.) <u>PHLEBOTHROMBOSIS</u>

Risk factors: 1. endothelial injury   2. slow blood flow   3. abnormal clotting
Trousseau's sign = migratory venous thrombosis, often a/w neoplasms

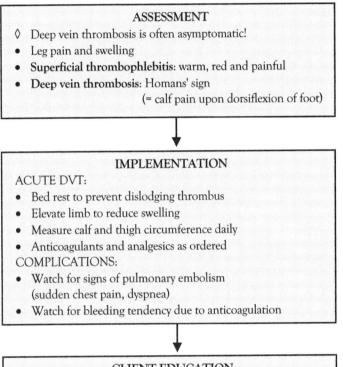

ASSESSMENT
◊ Deep vein thrombosis is often asymptomatic!
- Leg pain and swelling
- **Superficial thrombophlebitis:** warm, red and painful
- **Deep vein thrombosis:** Homans' sign
  (= calf pain upon dorsiflexion of foot)

IMPLEMENTATION
ACUTE DVT:
- Bed rest to prevent dislodging thrombus
- Elevate limb to reduce swelling
- Measure calf and thigh circumference daily
- Anticoagulants and analgesics as ordered
COMPLICATIONS:
- Watch for signs of pulmonary embolism
  (sudden chest pain, dyspnea)
- Watch for bleeding tendency due to anticoagulation

CLIENT EDUCATION
- Regular use of compression stockings to prevent DVT

RESPIRATORY
DISEASES

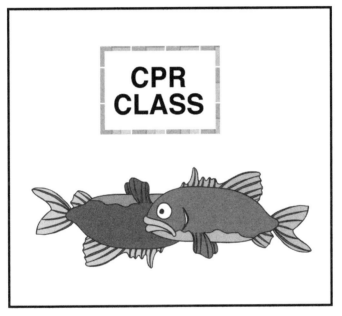

Gill-to-gill resuscitation

5.1.) PHYSIOLOGY

VC = vital capacity	- volume between maximal inspiration and maximal expiration - can be measured by spirometer - *decreased in COPD*
RV = residual volume	- volume left after maximal expiration - cannot be measured by spirometer - *increased in COPD*
TLC = total lung capacity	- vital capacity plus residual volume
FEV₁	- volume that can be expired during 1 second with maximal force - *important to monitor in asthma patients!*

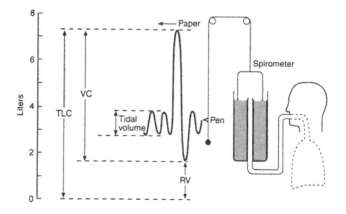

5.2) BREATHING PATTERNS

Biot respiration	- **episodes of apnea** alternating with regular breaths - due to CNS lesions
Cheyne Stokes respiration	- **waxing and waning** (hyperpnea ↔ apnea) - common at high altitude
Kussmaul respiration	- **hyperventilation:** deep, rapid, sighing - due to metabolic acidosis (e.g. diabetic coma)
breath odors	- **fruity:** ketoacidosis - **sweet, musty:** liver failure - **urine-like:** uremia, renal failure - **foul:** lung abscess, bronchiectasis
barrel chest	- **increased anterior-posterior chest diameter** - due to loss of lung elasticity - late stage of COPD
nasal flaring	- **respiratory distress** - important sign in infants *(they can't tell you!)*

5.3.) LUNG SOUNDS

crackles (rales & crepitations)	- rattling noises, usually during inspiration - movement of air through fluid-filled airways - **bronchitis, pneumonia, lung edema**
wheezing	- high-pitched musical quality - cannot be cleared by coughing - **bronchospasm, mucosal edema, asthma**
stridor	- loud, musical sound - usually inspiratory - **obstruction of larynx or trachea**

PULMONARY EDEMA AND IT'S CAUSES:

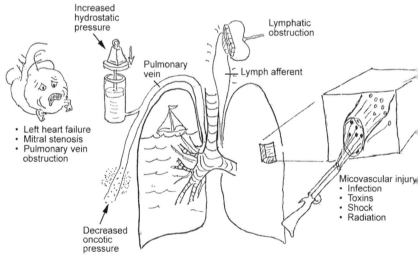

Increased hydrostatic pressure

Lymphatic obstruction

Pulmonary vein

Lymph afferent

- Left heart failure
- Mitral stenosis
- Pulmonary vein obstruction

Micovascular injury
- Infection
- Toxins
- Shock
- Radiation

Decreased oncotic pressure

From Zaher: *Pathology Made Ridiculously Simple*, MedMaster, 2007

74

5.4.) PULMONARY CARE PRINCIPLES

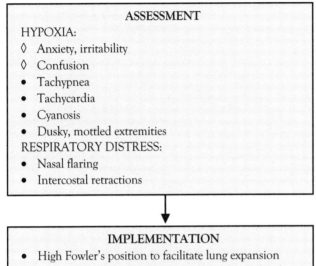

ASSESSMENT

HYPOXIA:
◊ Anxiety, irritability
◊ Confusion
• Tachypnea
• Tachycardia
• Cyanosis
• Dusky, mottled extremities

RESPIRATORY DISTRESS:
• Nasal flaring
• Intercostal retractions

IMPLEMENTATION
• High Fowler's position to facilitate lung expansion
• Pursed lip breathing to facilitate emptying of alveoli
• Administer O_2 as prescribed

OXYGEN DELIVERY SYSTEMS:

nasal cannula	- delivers low concentrations of O_2 - *useful for COPD clients (low O_2)*
Venturi mask	- most reliable and accurate - *useful for COPD clients (low O_2)*
simple mask	- delivers higher concentrations of O_2
non-rebreather mask	- delivers highest concentration of O_2

 Expect oxygen toxicity if >50% O_2 for more than 48 hours.

5.5.) PNEUMOTHORAX
Accumulation of air in pleural space → collapse of lung

ASSESSMENT
◊ Sudden sharp pain
◊ Shortness of breath
• Hypotension, shock
• Neck vein distension
• Absent breathing sounds over collapsed lung

IMPLEMENTATION
• Bed rest
• Monitor vital signs
• Oxygen as needed
THORACOSTOMY / CHEST TUBES:
• Encourage coughing <u>after</u> chest tube is placed
  (this facilitates lung expansion)
• Watch for air leak (bubbling)
• Do not reposition tube
• If tube dislodges, cover with gaze and call for help

client →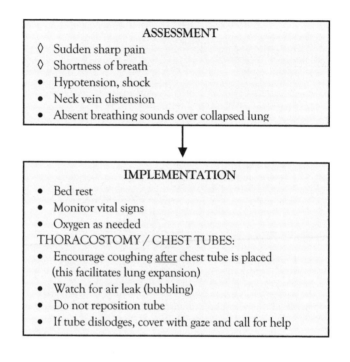

1 = collection bottle
2 = water seal bottle
3 = suction control bottle

COMMON CHEST TUBE PROBLEMS:

air leak	continuous bubbling in water seal bottle
kinks in tubing	no fluctuations in water seal with inspiration
insufficient suction	no bubbling in suction control bottle

5.6.) UPPER RESPIRATORY INFECTIONS

	MANAGEMENT
common cold	- no specific treatment
strep throat	- antibiotics are necessary to prevent complications (rheumatic fever and glomerulonephritis)
tonsillitis	- antibiotics - if recurrent: tonsillectomy - if peritonsillar abscess develops: need to drain plus parenteral antibiotics
influenza	- bed rest, analgesics - if fever persists or WBC > 12,000: suspect bacterial superinfection (→ antibiotics)
sinusitis	- most commonly involves maxillary sinus - nasal decongestants - antibiotics - purulent discharge should be send for culture - failure to resolve: hospitalization, drainage

Nasal decongestants should never be used for more than a few days!
(Mucosa becomes "drug dependent" resulting in stuffy nose as soon
as decongestant is withdrawn).

5.7.) PNEUMONIA

➢ **If community acquired:** probably due to *Streptococcus pneumoniae*
➢ **If hospital acquired:** Gram-negative bacilli, *Pseudomonas*, others...

TYPES:

BACTERIAL

bronchopneumonia
- patchy, peribronchial distribution
- more common in infants and elderly

lobar pneumonia
- diffuse involvement of entire lobe
- more common in middle age adults

ATYPICAL

viral or mycoplasma
- interstitial pneumonia
  (spares intra-alveolar spaces)

Mycoplasma pneumonia is common in young adults!

FUNGAL

Pneumocystis jirovecii
- only seen in immunocompromised patients
  (AIDS!)
- diffuse bilateral consolidation of lungs
- often presents with persistent, dry cough
- diagnosis: sputum

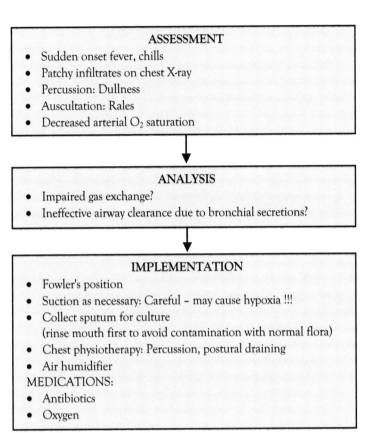

ASSESSMENT
- Sudden onset fever, chills
- Patchy infiltrates on chest X-ray
- Percussion: Dullness
- Auscultation: Rales
- Decreased arterial O_2 saturation

ANALYSIS
- Impaired gas exchange?
- Ineffective airway clearance due to bronchial secretions?

IMPLEMENTATION
- Fowler's position
- Suction as necessary: Careful – may cause hypoxia !!!
- Collect sputum for culture
  (rinse mouth first to avoid contamination with normal flora)
- Chest physiotherapy: Percussion, postural draining
- Air humidifier
MEDICATIONS:
- Antibiotics
- Oxygen

⁄ACCINATION RECOMMENDATIONS:

PNEUMOVAX (give once)	INFLUENZA (give every autumn)
- elderly > 65 years - clients with chronic illness [1]	- everyone above age 6 months !
- prior to splenectomy	- if client has fever, wait until fever is gone

[1] *COPD, HIV infection, congestive heart failure, diabetes mellitus*

5.8.) TUBERCULOSIS

Caused by mycobacterium tuberculosis – spread by droplets

primary	◊ usually asymptomatic • hilar lymphadenopathy • Ghon complex : calcified peripheral nodule plus calcified hilar lymph node
secondary (reactivation)	◊ fatigue • mild fever, weight loss • cough • multiple foci in apical areas of lung
generalized, miliary TBC (spread through blood)	• high fever, illness • pleurisy, pericarditis • meningitis • genitourinary involvement • bone and joint involvement

1. Tubercle (primary lesion)

Scar   Calcified Granuloma   Necrosis, Cavity

(reactivation)

2. Necrosis, Cavities

3. Systemic spread

ASSESSMENT

◊ Fatigue, weakness
- Weight loss
- Night sweats, low-grade fever
- Chest X-ray: early → Ghon complex
  late → cavities
- Positive sputum culture (acid fast bacilli)
- Positive tuberculin skin test

IMPLEMENTATION

- Assess respirations, breath sounds and vital signs
- Wear mask if patient is infectious (OSHA requirement)
- Watch for side effects of medications (see 23.3.)
MEDICATIONS = 4 DRUG REGIME:
- Isoniazid + Rifampin + Pyrazinamide + Ethambutol

CLIENT EDUCATION

- Avoid physical exertion
- Always cough or sneeze into tissue
- Client needs to understand that he is given multiple
  medications to prevent bacterial drug-resistance

 Multi drug-resistance is an ever-increasing problem !

INDICATIONS FOR TUBERCULIN SKIN TEST:
➢ Close contacts of persons with tuberculosis
➢ Immigrants from Africa, Asia, South America
➢ Residents of nursing homes etc.
➢ HIV positive clients

5.9.) CHRONIC OBSTR. PULMONARY DISEASE

- Group of diseases that obstruct pulmonary airflow.
- Many patients have combined elements of bronchitis, asthma and emphysema:

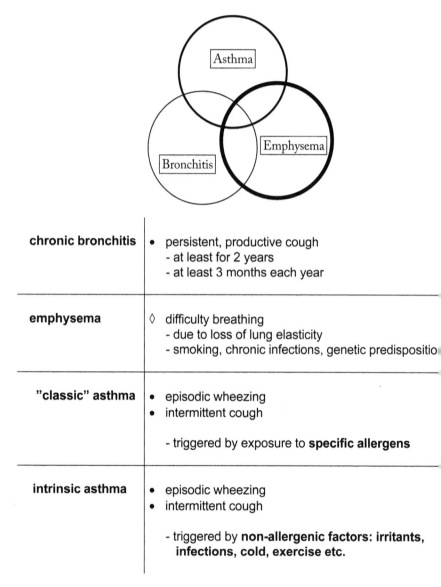

chronic bronchitis	• persistent, productive cough
	  - at least for 2 years
	  - at least 3 months each year

emphysema	◊ difficulty breathing
	  - due to loss of lung elasticity
	  - smoking, chronic infections, genetic predispositio▮

"classic" asthma	• episodic wheezing • intermittent cough - triggered by exposure to **specific allergens**

intrinsic asthma	• episodic wheezing
	• intermittent cough
	
	  - triggered by **non-allergenic factors: irritants,
	   infections, cold, exercise etc.**

5.10.) <u>CHRONIC BRONCHITIS</u>

COMPLICATIONS:
➤ **Atelectasis:** Shrunken, airless part of lung due to bronchial obstruction.
➤ **Bronchiectasis:** Irreversible dilation of bronchi due to chronic infection.

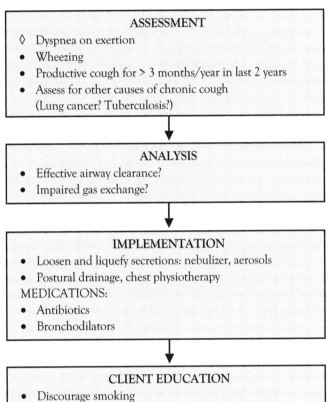

ASSESSMENT
◊ Dyspnea on exertion
• Wheezing
• Productive cough for > 3 months/year in last 2 years
• Assess for other causes of chronic cough
  (Lung cancer? Tuberculosis?)

ANALYSIS
• Effective airway clearance?
• Impaired gas exchange?

IMPLEMENTATION
• Loosen and liquefy secretions: nebulizer, aerosols
• Postural drainage, chest physiotherapy
MEDICATIONS:
• Antibiotics
• Bronchodilators

CLIENT EDUCATION
• Discourage smoking
• Avoid airway infections

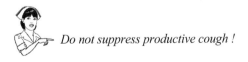

Do not suppress productive cough !

5.11.) <u>EMPHYSEMA</u>
Loss of lung elasticity → destruction of alveoli

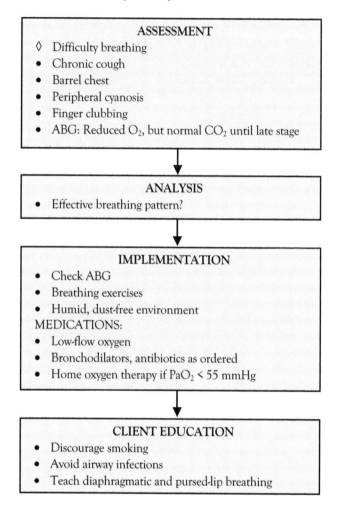

ASSESSMENT
- ◊ Difficulty breathing
- Chronic cough
- Barrel chest
- Peripheral cyanosis
- Finger clubbing
- ABG: Reduced O_2, but normal CO_2 until late stage

ANALYSIS
- Effective breathing pattern?

IMPLEMENTATION
- Check ABG
- Breathing exercises
- Humid, dust-free environment
MEDICATIONS:
- Low-flow oxygen
- Bronchodilators, antibiotics as ordered
- Home oxygen therapy if PaO_2 < 55 mmHg

CLIENT EDUCATION
- Discourage smoking
- Avoid airway infections
- Teach diaphragmatic and pursed-lip breathing

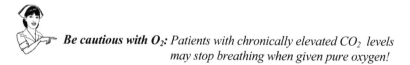

Be cautious with O_2: *Patients with chronically elevated CO_2 levels may stop breathing when given pure oxygen!*

5.12.) ASTHMA

Hyperresponsiveness of airways → sudden narrowing and obstruction

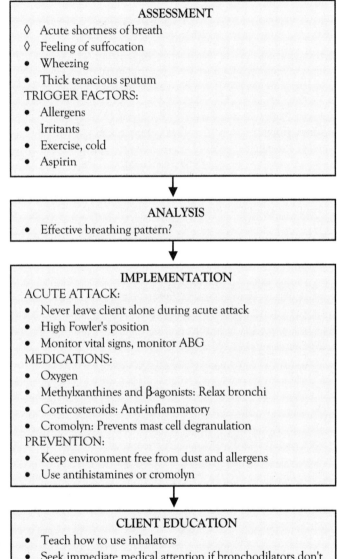

ASSESSMENT
◊ Acute shortness of breath
◊ Feeling of suffocation
• Wheezing
• Thick tenacious sputum
TRIGGER FACTORS:
• Allergens
• Irritants
• Exercise, cold
• Aspirin

ANALYSIS
• Effective breathing pattern?

IMPLEMENTATION
ACUTE ATTACK:
• Never leave client alone during acute attack
• High Fowler's position
• Monitor vital signs, monitor ABG
MEDICATIONS:
• Oxygen
• Methylxanthines and β-agonists: Relax bronchi
• Corticosteroids: Anti-inflammatory
• Cromolyn: Prevents mast cell degranulation
PREVENTION:
• Keep environment free from dust and allergens
• Use antihistamines or cromolyn

CLIENT EDUCATION
• Teach how to use inhalators
• Seek immediate medical attention if bronchodilators don't stop attack

5.13.) <u>RESTRICTIVE LUNG DISEASES</u>

Increased lung stiffness → limited respiration and gas exchange

	EXAMPLES
pneumoconiosis (inorganic substances)	- quartz - coal dust - asbestos
pulmonary fibrosis (often drug induced)	- bleomycin - alkylating agents - oxygen therapy
hypersensitivity pneumonitis (allergy)	- farmer's lung - cotton worker's lung - pigeon breeder's lung

---

ASBESTOS RELATED DISEASES:
➤ **Asbestosis** (chronic interstitial fibrosis)
➤ **Lung cancer** = 5~100fold risk

Smoking multiplies risk of asbestos exposure !!!

5.14.) SHOCK LUNG (ARDS)

Pulmonary edema caused by increased permeability of alveolar capillaries

MANY CAUSES OF ALVEOLAR INJURY:

➤ Inhalation of smoke or toxic chemicals
➤ Aspiration of gastric content
➤ Pneumonia (viral or bacterial), sepsis
➤ Pancreatitis
➤ Major surgery
➤ Shock (any cause)

ASSESSMENT

◊ Dyspnea
• Rapid shallow breathing
• Intercostal retractions during inspiration
• Auscultation: Crackles and rhonchi
• Cough: clear, frothy sputum
• Decrease in arterial O_2 despite oxygen therapy
• Hypotension, shock

IMPLEMENTATION

• High Fowler's position
• Monitor ventilator, ABG and vital signs
MEDICATIONS:
• Oxygen
• Positive airway pressure if necessary (PEEP)
• Diuretics

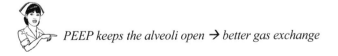

PEEP keeps the alveoli open → better gas exchange

5.15.) <u>LUNG CANCER</u>

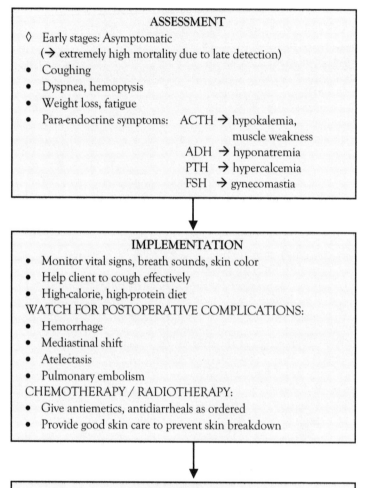

ASSESSMENT
◊ Early stages: Asymptomatic
  (➜ extremely high mortality due to late detection)
- Coughing
- Dyspnea, hemoptysis
- Weight loss, fatigue
- Para-endocrine symptoms: ACTH ➜ hypokalemia,
                                        muscle weakness
                            ADH ➜ hyponatremia
                            PTH ➜ hypercalcemia
                            FSH ➜ gynecomastia

IMPLEMENTATION
- Monitor vital signs, breath sounds, skin color
- Help client to cough effectively
- High-calorie, high-protein diet
WATCH FOR POSTOPERATIVE COMPLICATIONS:
- Hemorrhage
- Mediastinal shift
- Atelectasis
- Pulmonary embolism
CHEMOTHERAPY / RADIOTHERAPY:
- Give antiemetics, antidiarrheals as ordered
- Provide good skin care to prevent skin breakdown

CLIENT EDUCATION
- Most common cause of cancer <u>death</u> in US !
- Smoking causes >90% of lung cancers !

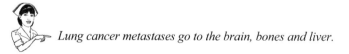

Lung cancer metastases go to the brain, bones and liver.

GASTROINTESTINAL DISEASES

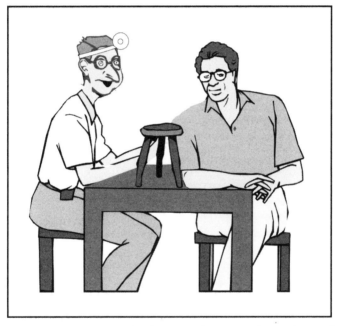

"Sorry, that's not why I meant by a stool specimen."

6.1.) <u>ALTERATION IN NUTRITION</u>

Body mass index = weight / height^2 (normal is 20~25 kg/m^2)
1. convert pound to kg: 1 lb. = 0.453 kg
2. convert feet to meter: 1 ft. = 0.305 m
3. convert inches to meter: 1 in. = 0.025 m

<u>EXAMPLE</u>: "Client is 5'10 tall and weighs 180 lbs."
1. weight (180 lbs.) = 81.5 kg
2. height (5 ft. +10 in.) = 1.525 + 0.25 m = 1.78 m
3. BMI = 81.5 / (1.78 · 1.78) = 81.5/3.17 = 25.7
→ client is slightly overweight

<u>MARASMUS (=SEVERE MALNUTRITION)</u>
➤ Watch for electrolyte imbalance
➤ Do not refeed too rapidly !

<u>OBESITY</u>
➤ "Yo-yo dieting" may be a/w increased risk for coronary artery disease
➤ Surgery (gastroplasty, gastric bypass) only for severe obesity (BMI > 40)

<u>ANOREXIA NERVOSA</u>
➤ Psychotherapy often required
➤ Restore normal eating pattern / caloric intake
➤ Force-feed in life-threatening situations

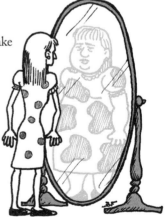

"I look too fat..."

6.2.) MOUTH: SIGNS & SYMPTOMS

bleeding gums	Vit. C deficiency
glossitis, cheilosis	Vit. B2 deficiency
smooth beefy red tongue	Vit. B12 deficiency
strawberry tongue	scarlet fever
Koplik's spots (small red spots with white center on buccal mucosa)	measles
thrush (white, removable plaques)	*Candida albicans*

6.3.) GI BLEEDING

SIGNS & SYMPTOMS:

hematemesis	• vomiting bright red blood **(rapid bleed)** • vomiting "coffee-ground" **(slow bleed)**
melena	• black, tarry stool • source: **upper GI**, or small bowels
hematochezia	• bright red blood in stool • source: **lower GI** (or upper GI if massive)

MEDICAL CAUSES:

UPPER GI	LOWER GI	UPPER & LOWER GI

- esophageal varices
 	
- gastritis
- gastric ulcer
- duodenal ulcer
	- hemorrhoids
	- anal fissure
	
	- diverticulosis
	- inflammatory bowel
	  disease
	- intussusception
		- neoplasms
		- angiodysplasias
		  (Osler's disease)

6.4.) UPPER ABDOMINAL PAIN

reflux esophagitis	◊ burning substernal pain ◊ **after meals, at night** ◊ may radiate to left arm!
gastric ulcer	◊ steady, gnawing epigastric pain ◊ **worsened by food**
duodenal ulcer	◊ steady, gnawing epigastric pain ◊ typically awakens patient around 1:00 am ◊ **relieved by food**
perforated peptic ulcer	◊ severe epigastric pain ◊ may radiate to back or shoulders • peritoneal signs
cholecystitis	◊ cramp-like epigastric pain ◊ may radiate to tip of right scapula • Murphy's sign
acute pancreatitis	◊ severe, boring abdominal pain ◊ often radiates to back • peritoneal signs (rebound tenderness, abdominal rigidity)

6.5.) <u>ESOPHAGITIS</u>

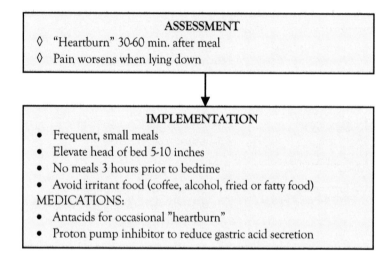

ASSESSMENT
◊ "Heartburn" 30-60 min. after meal
◊ Pain worsens when lying down

IMPLEMENTATION
- Frequent, small meals
- Elevate head of bed 5-10 inches
- No meals 3 hours prior to bedtime
- Avoid irritant food (coffee, alcohol, fried or fatty food)

MEDICATIONS:
- Antacids for occasional "heartburn"
- Proton pump inhibitor to reduce gastric acid secretion

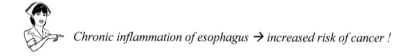

Chronic inflammation of esophagus → increased risk of cancer !

6.6.) <u>HIATAL HERNIA</u>

➤ **Sliding hernia:** gastroesophageal junction and part of stomach slide upwards
➤ **Paraesophageal hernia:** part of stomach turns adjacent to esophagus

---

ASSESSMENT
◊ Often asymptomatic
◊ Heartburn
◊ Regurgitation of food
• Diagnosis: Chest X-ray or barium swallow

IMPLEMENTATION
• If asymptomatic → no treatment necessary
• Small frequent meals
• Elevate head of bed to reduce acid reflux
• Avoid activities that increase abdominal pressure:
  (lifting heavy objects, bending over etc.)

<u>TYPES OF HERNIAS</u>:

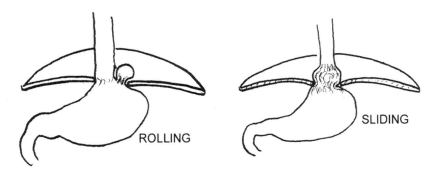

From Zaher: *Pathology Made Ridiculously Simple*, MedMaster, 2007

95

6.7.) ESOPHAGEAL VARICES

Liver cirrhosis → elevated portal vein pressure → esophageal varices

ASSESSMENT
◊ History of alcohol abuse (liver cirrhosis)
• **Hematemesis** = vomiting blood
• **Melena** = black, tarry stools
• Signs of shock if bleeding is severe

IMPLEMENTATION
• Watch for hemorrhage, hypotension, signs of shock
• Monitor vital signs if acute bleeding
• Watch for signs of hepatic encephalopathy
• Assist with Sengstaken tube

Sengstaken tube (to compress varices):
➢ Monitor bleeding in gastric drainage
➢ Watch for signs of asphyxiation
➢ Watch for tube displacement

6.8.) <u>GASTRITIS</u>

Inflammation of gastric mucosa

acute gastritis (erosive)	- acute hemorrhagic lesions - stress ulcers - aspirin, NSAIDs - alcohol
chronic gastritis type A **(non-erosive)**	**- autoimmune gastritis** - involves body and fundus - pernicious anemia [1]
chronic gastritis type B **(non-erosive)**	**- infectious gastritis** - involves body and antrum - *H. pylori*

[1] *treatment: monthly, lifelong IM injections of vit. B12*

ASSESSMENT
◊ Nausea, anorexia
◊ Sour taste in mouth
• Belching
• Cramping, pain

IMPLEMENTATION
• Watch for signs of GI bleeding ("coffee-ground" vomit)
• CBC if suspected pernicious anemia
MEDICATIONS:
• Antacids
• Proton pump inhibitors to reduce acid secretion
• Antibiotics to eradicate *H. pylori*

6.9.) PEPTIC ULCER DISEASE

gastric ulcer	- normal or decreased acid production - decreased mucosal resistance - chronic NSAID use • Pain gets worse after meals
duodenal ulcer	- increased acid production - *H. pylori* • Pain typically relieved by meals

---

ASSESSMENT
◊ Gnawing, burning epigastric pain
• Vomiting
• GI bleeding → anemia
• Diagnosis: - Upper GI series or endoscopy
           - Test for presence of *Helicobacter pylori*

↓

IMPLEMENTATION
• Watch for signs of bleeding -"coffee-ground" vomit
                             - tarry stools
• Avoid irritating food
• Avoid cigarette smoking
• Avoid aspirin, NSAIDs and steroids
MEDICATIONS:
• Proton pump inhibitors
• Antibiotics to eradicate *H. pylori*

Gastric resection very rare nowadays due to more effective drugs, especially the use of antibiotics to eradicate H. pylori

6.10.) LIVER: SIGNS & SYMPTOMS

	DUE TO:
jaundice	- diminished bilirubin secretion
fetor hepaticus	- sulfur compounds produced by intestinal bacteria, not cleared by liver
spider angiomas palmar erythema gynecomastia	- elevated estrogen levels
ecchymoses (easy bruising)	- decreased synthesis of clotting factors
xanthomas (yellow skin plaques / nodules)	- elevated cholesterol levels
hypoglycemia	- decreased liver glycogen stores - decreased liver glucose production
splenomegaly	- portal hypertension
encephalopathy asterixis (hand-flapping tremor)	- portosystemic shunt (digestive products bypass liver and are not detoxified)

99

6.11.) LIVER: LAB DATA

AST (GOT) ↑	- **hepatitis** - also elevated in acute MI
gamma-GT ↑	- **alcoholism** - persistent liver cell damage
direct bilirubin ↑ (conjugated)	- biliary obstruction - drug induced cholestasis
indirect bilirubin ↑ (unconjugated)	- hemolytic anemia - physiologic jaundice of the newborn
HBs-Ag	- earliest marker of hepatitis B
HBe-Ag	- indicates infective state (hepatitis B)

6.12.) JAUNDICE

Skin looks yellow if serum bilirubin > 2 mg/dL

prehepatic	hemolysis: - sickle cell anemia - hemolytic anemias (antibodies against RBCs)
hepatic	hepatitis: - impaired conjugation of bilirubin by liver cells
posthepatic	cholestasis: - impaired excretion by liver (estrogens, some drugs) - bile duct obstruction

6.13.) DRUG INDUCED LIVER DISEASE

estrogens **chlorpromazine**	- reversible cholestasis
ethanol	- fatty liver - cirrhosis
acetaminophen **carbon tetrachloride**	- acute liver cell necrosis
estrogens	- hepatocellular adenoma (benign)
aflatoxin **hepatitis B and C**	- hepatocellular carcinoma

 Acetaminophen overdose is most dangerous in infants (immature liver) and alcoholics (damaged liver).

6.14.) <u>LIVER CIRRHOSIS</u>

ASSESSMENT

◊ Fatigue
◊ Anorexia
◊ Nausea
◊ Itchy skin
● Jaundice
● Spider angiomas
● Palmar erythema
● Nosebleeds, GI bleeds, bruises
● Ascites
● Esophageal varices → risk of severe bleeding!
● CNS: lethargy
LAB:
● Elevated AST, ALT, bilirubin, ammonia

ANALYSIS

● Altered thought process?
● Nutritional status?
● Bleeding risk?
● Skin integrity?

IMPLEMENTATION

● Check skin, gums and stool for bleeding
● Avoid aspirin
● Monitor weight
● Monitor abdominal circumference
● If ascites interferes with breathing → high Fowler's position
DIET:
● High-carbohydrate, high-caloric diet, vitamins
  (low-protein diet if client has hepatic encephalopathy)
● Provide counseling if client abuses alcohol

6.15.) HEPATITIS

A	contaminated water/food raw shellfish	- **fecal/oral** - 2~6 weeks incubation - 0% become chronic
B	blood transfusions sexual contact	- **parenteral** - 2~6 months incubation - 10% become chronic
C	blood transfusions sexual contact	- **parenteral** - 1~2 months incubation - 50% chronic
D	only in patients with hepatitis B	- **parenteral**
E		- **fecal oral** - mainly in Southeast Asia

Risk from blood transfusions about 1:50,000
Hepatitic C is most serious (high risk of chronic cirrhosis)

ISOLATION OF INFECTIOUS CLIENT:
➤ Required if client has hepatitis A or E and fecal incontinence
➤ Required if client has hepatitis B or C and is bleeding

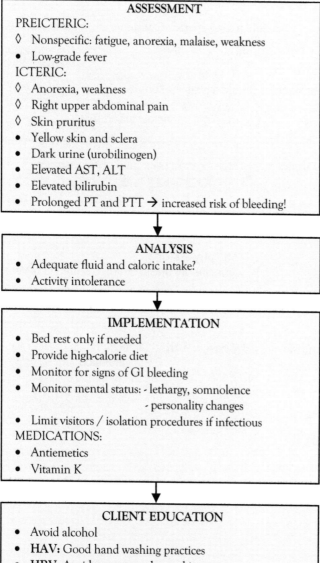

ASSESSMENT

PREICTERIC:
- ◊ Nonspecific: fatigue, anorexia, malaise, weakness
- • Low-grade fever

ICTERIC:
- ◊ Anorexia, weakness
- ◊ Right upper abdominal pain
- ◊ Skin pruritus
- • Yellow skin and sclera
- • Dark urine (urobilinogen)
- • Elevated AST, ALT
- • Elevated bilirubin
- • Prolonged PT and PTT → increased risk of bleeding!

ANALYSIS
- • Adequate fluid and caloric intake?
- • Activity intolerance

IMPLEMENTATION
- • Bed rest only if needed
- • Provide high-calorie diet
- • Monitor for signs of GI bleeding
- • Monitor mental status: - lethargy, somnolence
                           - personality changes
- • Limit visitors / isolation procedures if infectious

MEDICATIONS:
- • Antiemetics
- • Vitamin K

CLIENT EDUCATION
- • Avoid alcohol
- • **HAV:** Good hand washing practices
- • **HBV:** Avoid unprotected sexual intercourse
        Avoid sharing of needles

6.16.) GALLBLADDER

➢ Cholelithiasis = presence of gallstones in the gallbladder

cholelithiasis	usually asymptomatic (70%) may cause biliary colic (20%) may cause cholecystitis (10%)
biliary colic	- steady, cramplike pain in epigastrium - pain <u>subsides over 30~60 min.</u>
cholecystitis	- steady, cramplike pain in epigastrium - **Murphy's sign** (inspiratory arrest during palpation of liver margin) - pain <u>does not subside spontaneously</u>
cholangitis	**Charcot's triad** : 1. biliary pain 2. jaundice 3. fever

 Patients with asymptomatic gallstones do not require surgery.

6.17.) CHOLECYSTITIS

Usually due to stone obstructing gallbladder duct

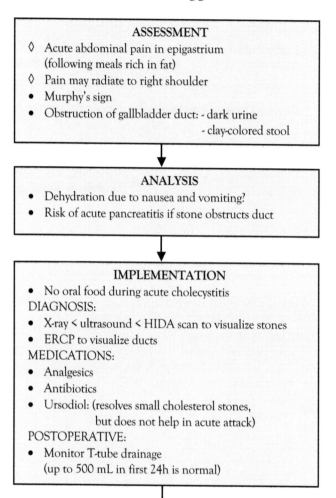

ASSESSMENT
◊ Acute abdominal pain in epigastrium
(following meals rich in fat)
◊ Pain may radiate to right shoulder
• Murphy's sign
• Obstruction of gallbladder duct: - dark urine
  - clay-colored stool

ANALYSIS
• Dehydration due to nausea and vomiting?
• Risk of acute pancreatitis if stone obstructs duct

IMPLEMENTATION
• No oral food during acute cholecystitis
DIAGNOSIS:
• X-ray < ultrasound < HIDA scan to visualize stones
• ERCP to visualize ducts
MEDICATIONS:
• Analgesics
• Antibiotics
• Ursodiol: (resolves small cholesterol stones,
  but does not help in acute attack)
POSTOPERATIVE:
• Monitor T-tube drainage
  (up to 500 mL in first 24h is normal)

CLIENT EDUCATION
• Reduce dietary fat and cholesterol intake

6.18.) PANCREATITIS

	ACUTE PANCREATITIS	CHRONIC PANCREATITIS
causes	alcohol abuse cholelithiasis	alcohol abuse rarely due to cholelithiasis
features	elevated lipase, amylase	pancreatic calcifications
	mortality rate ~ 10%	pancreatic insufficiency: - endocrine → diabetes mellitus - exocrine → maldigestion [1]

[1] *client requires dietary enzyme supplements: lipase, amylase, protease*

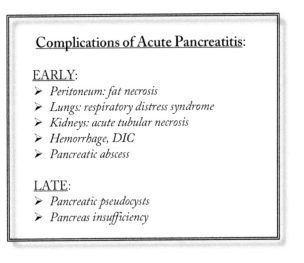

Complications of Acute Pancreatitis:

EARLY:
➤ *Peritoneum: fat necrosis*
➤ *Lungs: respiratory distress syndrome*
➤ *Kidneys: acute tubular necrosis*
➤ *Hemorrhage, DIC*
➤ *Pancreatic abscess*

LATE:
➤ *Pancreatic pseudocysts*
➤ *Pancreas insufficiency*

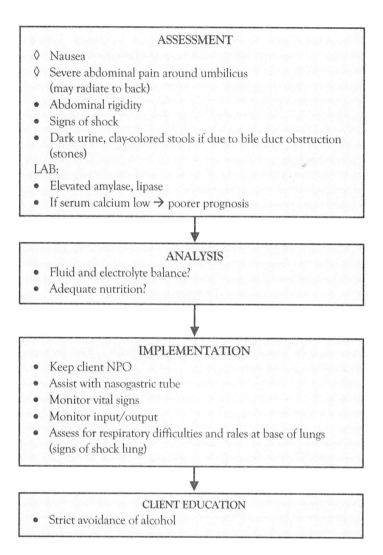

ASSESSMENT

◊ Nausea
◊ Severe abdominal pain around umbilicus
  (may radiate to back)
- Abdominal rigidity
- Signs of shock
- Dark urine, clay-colored stools if due to bile duct obstruction
  (stones)

LAB:
- Elevated amylase, lipase
- If serum calcium low → poorer prognosis

ANALYSIS

- Fluid and electrolyte balance?
- Adequate nutrition?

IMPLEMENTATION

- Keep client NPO
- Assist with nasogastric tube
- Monitor vital signs
- Monitor input/output
- Assess for respiratory difficulties and rales at base of lungs
  (signs of shock lung)

CLIENT EDUCATION

- Strict avoidance of alcohol

6.19.) MALDIGESTION

MALDIGESTION	MALABSORPTION
dysfunction of pancreas - chronic pancreatitis - cystic fibrosis **lack of specific enzymes** - lactase deficiency	**dysfunction of small bowel** - short bowel syndrome - bacterial overgrowth - celiac disease - tropical sprue

lack of bile salts
- biliary cirrhosis
- resected terminal ileum
- bacterial overgrowth

 Diarrhea often leads to transient lactase deficiency:
Teach client to avoid milk when having diarrhea of any cause.

6.20.) DIARRHEA

secretory	• large volume watery stools
	• persists with fasting
	
	   - cholera
	   - dysentery

osmotic	• bulky, greasy stools
	• improves with fasting
	
	   - lactase deficiency
	   - pancreatic insufficiency
	   - short bowel syndrome

inflammatory	• frequent but small stools
	• blood and/or pus
	
	   - inflammatory bowel disease
	   - irradiation
	   - shigella, amebiasis

dysmotility	• diarrhea alternating with constipation
	
	   - irritable bowel syndrome
	   - diabetes mellitus

6.21.) LOWER ABDOMINAL PAIN

appendicitis	◊ vague periumbilical pain, nausea ◊ later localizes to lower right quadrant • perforation: high fever and leukocytosis
diverticulitis	◊ elderly patients ◊ steady pain ◊ localized to lower left quadrant • "left sided appendicitis"
inflammatory bowel disease	◊ chronic, cramping pain • diarrhea, blood and pus in stool
intestinal obstruction	• hyperactive bowel sounds
intestinal infarction	• absent bowel sounds • gross or occult blood in stool

6.22.) <u>APPENDICITIS</u>

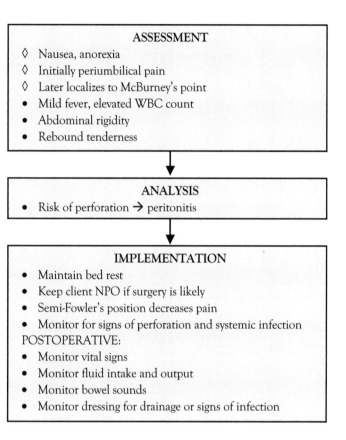

ASSESSMENT
◊ Nausea, anorexia
◊ Initially periumbilical pain
◊ Later localizes to McBurney's point
● Mild fever, elevated WBC count
● Abdominal rigidity
● Rebound tenderness

ANALYSIS
● Risk of perforation → peritonitis

IMPLEMENTATION
● Maintain bed rest
● Keep client NPO if surgery is likely
● Semi-Fowler's position decreases pain
● Monitor for signs of perforation and systemic infection
POSTOPERATIVE:
● Monitor vital signs
● Monitor fluid intake and output
● Monitor bowel sounds
● Monitor dressing for drainage or signs of infection

Do not apply heat to abdomen. Do not apply enemas and avoid unnecessary palpation (risk of rupture) !

6.23.) <u>DIVERTICULITIS</u>

Diverticula = bulging pouches of mucosa through surrounding muscle

 Diverticulosis: *Presence of diverticula (often asymptomatic).*
Diverticulitis: *Inflammation of diverticula.*

ASSESSMENT
- ◊ Pain in lower left quadrant
- ◊ May be relieved by bowel movement
- ◊ Bowel irregularities
- • Rectal bleeding
- • Mild fever
- • Elevated WBC
- • Diagnosis: Barium enema
  - Sigmoidoscopy, colonoscopy

IMPLEMENTATION
- • NPO if peritonitis or massive bleeding
- • Liquid or soft diet during acute phase
- • High fiber and bulk-forming diet after pain subsides
- • Stool softeners
- • Temporary colostomy necessary if: perforation, peritonitis
  - or obstruction

POSTOPERATIVE
- • Monitor vital signs
- • Monitor fluid intake and output
- • Watch for bleeding: hematocrit and hemoglobin
- • Watch for signs of infection: pus or foul odor

6.24.) HEMORRHOIDS
Varicosities of anal and rectal veins

Predisposing factors:
➢ Hereditary
➢ Chronic constipation
➢ Pregnancy
➢ Liver cirrhosis

ASSESSMENT
◊ Rectal pain and itching
• Bleeding (bright red blood on stool)

IMPLEMENTATION
• Warm "Sitz baths" to ease pain and swelling
• Stool softeners, high fiber diet
• Avoid straining
• Surgery: Ligation, sclerotherapy or surgical excision
TOPICAL MEDICATIONS:
• Anti-inflammatory: hydrocortisone cream
• Astringents: witch hazel cream ("Preparation H")
POSTOPERATIVE:
• Watch for rectal bleeding
• Good anal hygiene – keep dry

6.25.) <u>INFLAMMATORY BOWEL DISEASE</u>

CROHN'S DISEASE *(regional enteritis)*	**ULCERATIVE COLITIS**
◊ cramping abdominal pain • fever, anorexia, weight loss	◊ less abdominal pain • more bloody diarrhea
<u>PATHOLOGY</u> - transmural thickening - granulomas - usually involves ileum - rectum often spared - affects several bowel segments	<u>PATHOLOGY</u> - mucosal ulceration - begins at rectum and progresses - towards ileocecal junction - limited to colon (but may involve terminal ileum)
<u>COMPLICATIONS</u> - perianal disease - fistulas - perforation	<u>COMPLICATIONS</u> - increased risk for colon carcinoma
<u>OUTCOME</u> - many patients will have disease recurrence a few years after surgery.	<u>OUTCOME</u> - surgery is curative.

The causes of Crohn's disease and ulcerative colitis are unknown.
These patients often have additional chronic inflammations such
as sacroiliitis, iritis or conjunctivitis.

A) Ulcerative Colitis:

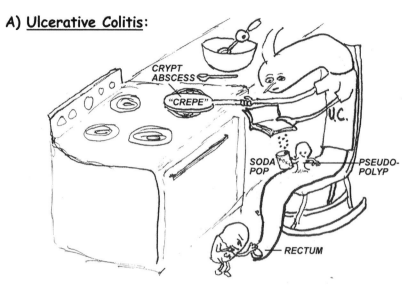

B) Crohn's Disease:

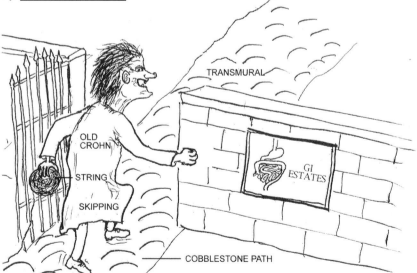

From Zaher: *Pathology Made Ridiculously Simple*, MedMaster, 2007

ASSESSMENT

◊ Abdominal pain and cramping
  (may mimic appendicitis)
◊ Malaise, weakness
◊ Anxiety
• Chronic diarrhea with blood, pus or mucus
• Fever, elevated WBC count
• Weight loss
• Diagnosis: Barium enema, endoscopy with biopsy

ANALYSIS

• Adequate nutritional intake?
• Fluid and electrolyte balance?

IMPLEMENTATION

• Watch for dehydration
• Monitor stool frequency and consistency
• Monitor hemoglobin and hematocrit
• Watch for signs of gastrointestinal obstruction
• Provide psychological support and counseling
DIET:
• Acute phase: bowel rest → NPO → low-residue diet
• Low-fat diet for steatorrhea
• Avoid milk (lactose deficiency of chronic diarrhea)
MEDICATIONS:
• Sulfasalazine
• Steroids
SURGERY:
• indicated if perforation, obstruction or cancer develops

6.26.) INTESTINAL OBSTRUCTION

Mechanical obstruction ➜ ischemia ➜ necrosis ➜ shock ➜ death

Mechanical obstruction:
➢ Due to adhesions, tumors, volvulus (twisting)
➢ Increased bowel sounds

Paralytic ileus:
➢ Due to toxins, uremia, infections or postoperative
➢ Absent bowel sounds

ASSESSMENT
◊ Nausea
◊ Colicky pain
• Constipation
• Vomiting
  (fecal vomiting in severe lower bowel obstruction)
• Diagnosis: - abdominal film: intestinal gas
             - endoscopy

IMPLEMENTATION
• Maintain NPO
• Monitor vital signs
• Turn client supine ↔ prone
  (helps passing flatus and relief abdominal pressure)
• Monitor patency of decompression tube
POSTOPERATIVE:
• Encourage coughing, turning, deep breathing
• Monitor bowel sounds (return of peristalsis)

Upper intestinal obstruction:
- risk of metabolic alkalosis due to loss of gastric acid
Lower intestinal obstruction:
- risk of metabolic acidosis due to loss of alkaline fluid

119

6.27.) PERITONITIS

acute inflammation of peritoneum

bacterial	- perforated duodenal ulcer - ruptured appendicitis - volvulus (twisting of bowel → strangulation, obstruction) - abdominal trauma
chemical	- pancreatitis - perforated gastric ulcer

Mortality dramatically decreased with antibiotics !

ASSESSMENT
◊ Constant, intense, diffuse abdominal pain
◊ Nausea
◊ Weakness
• Abdominal rigidity
• Absent bowel sounds
• Signs and symptoms of shock
• Diagnostic paracentesis: cytology, bacterial culture

↓

IMPLEMENTATION
• NPO to reduce peristalsis
• Monitor vital signs
• Maintain bed rest
• Semi-Fowler's position
• IV electrolytes and antibiotics as ordered

6.28.) <u>COLORECTAL CANCER</u>

➤ Second most common cancer in US
➤ 5 year mortality about 50%
➤ Early diagnosis significantly improves survival

 Ask client about any change in bowel habits or form of stool !
Suspect cancer in all elderly with anemia and occult rectal bleeding !

ASSESSMENT
◊ Vague abdominal discomfort
◊ Nausea, loss of appetite
◊ Weakness, fatigue
◊ Family history of colorectal cancer
• Ribbon- or pencil-shaped stools
• Black tarry stools
• Anemia
• Signs of intestinal obstruction
• Diagnosis: sigmoidoscopy, colonoscopy with biopsy
            CEA blood test to detect recurrence after surgery

---

IMPLEMENTATION
• Monitor intake and output
• Monitor consistency and color of stool
• Prepare client for surgery
COLOSTOMY CARE:
• Remove pouch when about $^1/_3$ full
• Cleanse stoma with soft cloth and water or mild soap
• Dry skin thoroughly before applying pouch
• Use skin barrier powder or paste to protect from fecal drainage
• Irrigation of stoma: be gentle – never force catheter
• Allow client to verbalize feelings about colostomy

UROGENITAL
DISEASES

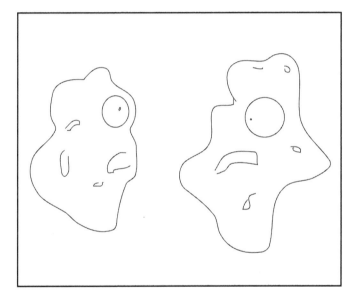

"Don't worry my dear, erectile dysfunction isn't the end of the World, especially if you're an ameba."

7.1.) PHYSIOLOGY

glomeruli 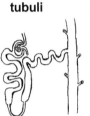	*20% of renal plasma flow is filtered through the glomeruli:* - electrolytes, sugars, amino acids - water soluble toxins and drugs
tubuli	*Absorption:* - most of the water filtered by glomeruli is reabsorbed - most electrolytes, sugars and amino acids are reabsorbed *Secretion:* - some drugs and toxins are secreted by the tubuli - acids (H^+) are secreted by the tubuli

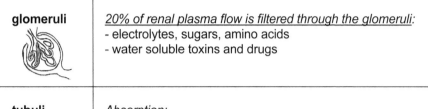

➢ Damage to glomeruli (glomerulonephritis):
  Albumin is filtered and lost with the urine → nephrotic syndrome
➢ Damage to tubuli (acute renal failure):
  Electrolyte imbalances
  Metabolic acidosis

RENAL HORMONES:

renin	*if urine flow at the tubuli is low, the kidneys release renin:* - renin increases aldosterone levels → increased water and sodium reabsorption - renin increases angiotensin levels → increased blood pressu
erythropoietin	*if oxygen is low, the kidneys produce erythropoietin:* - stimulates red blood cell production in bone marrow

➢ Arteriosclerosis of renal artery → renin release → high blood pressure
➢ Patients with chronic renal failure often have anemia (lack of erythropoietin).

7.2.) ASSESSMENT: URINE

pH	- **acidic**: high protein diet ketoacidosis (diabetes, starvation) - **alkaline**: urinary tract infections
specific gravity	**low = dilute urine:** - tubular defect - lack of ADH (diabetes insipidus) - polydipsia: client drinks too much
reducing sugars	glucose, fructose, galactose
ketones	dieting starvation diabetic ketoacidosis

7.3.) <u>LOWER URINARY TRACT INFECTIONS</u>
(cystitis and/or urethritis)

➤ More common in women due to shorter length of urethra.
➤ Indwelling catheter → high risk

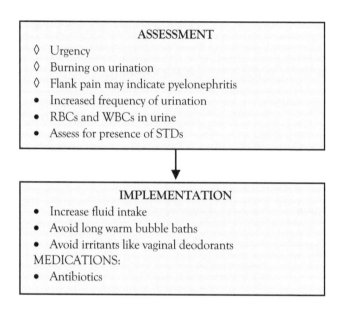

ASSESSMENT
◊ Urgency
◊ Burning on urination
◊ Flank pain may indicate pyelonephritis
• Increased frequency of urination
• RBCs and WBCs in urine
• Assess for presence of STDs

IMPLEMENTATION
• Increase fluid intake
• Avoid long warm bubble baths
• Avoid irritants like vaginal deodorants
MEDICATIONS:
• Antibiotics

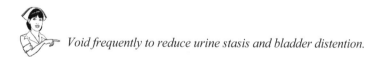

Void frequently to reduce urine stasis and bladder distention.

7.4.) KIDNEY STONES
Precipitation of calcium phosphates, urate, or cystine

	DIETARY RECOMMENDATIONS
calcium stones	increase acid-ash foods to **acidify urine**: - *cranberry juice, prunes* - *meat*
cystine stones	increases alkaline-ash foods to **alkalinize urine**: - *vegetables*
uric acid stones	avoid food high in **purines**: - *sardines, scallops, organ meat*

ASSESSMENT
◊ Severe suprapubic or pelvic or flank pain
◊ Chills
• Increased frequency of urination
• Hematuria, pyuria
• Diagnosis: IVP, Ultrasound, Urinalysis

↓

ANALYSIS
• Risk of infection and injury
• Adequate urinary elimination?

↓

IMPLEMENTATION
• Increase fluid intake
• Monitor intake/output and urine pH
• Harvest all solid material for urinalysis
• Prepare client for surgery or shock wave lithotripsy
MEDICATIONS:
• Analgesics as needed

127

7.5.) KIDNEYS: LAB DATA

serum BUN ↑	- **renal failure** - dehydration - high protein intake
serum creatinine ↑	- **renal failure** - diet (meat...)
creatinine clearance ↓	- most sensitive indicator of renal failure
serum uric acid ↑	- **gout** - **leukemia, metastatic cancer** client during chemotherapy

---

Instructions for 24h urine collection:
1. Void at 8^{00} am, then discard
2. Collect all urine until end of 24h period (8^{00} am next morning)
3. Keep on ice

7.6.) <u>GLOMERULONEPHRITIS</u>
Damage to glomerular membrane – due to antibodies or immune complexes

NEPHRITIC SYNDROME	NEPHROTIC SYNDROME
• hematuria • RBC casts	• proteinuria • hypoalbuminemia • hyperlipidemia • edema • puffy face

---

ASSESSMENT
◊ Weakness, fatigue
• Fluid retention → periorbital edema
• Hypertension
• Hematuria, Proteinuria

↓

ANALYSIS
• Risk of chronic renal failure

↓

IMPLEMENTATION
• Monitor intake and output closely, weigh daily
• Watch for signs of acute renal failure: oliguria, azotemia
DIET:
• High-protein diet for <u>nephrotic</u> syndrome
• Low-protein diet if renal failure develops
• Low-sodium
• Restrict fluids
MEDICATIONS:
• Diuretics and antihypertensives
• Glucocorticoids depending on biopsy result

Acute nephritic syndrome in children and young adults often follows streptococcal infection (check ASLO titer).

129

7.7.) ACUTE RENAL FAILURE

prerenal causes	**1. low cardiac output (shock)**
	
	2. hypovolemia
	  - hemorrhage
	  - burns
	  - sequestration
	
	3. systemic vasodilation
	  - sepsis
	  - anaphylaxis

renal causes	**1. acute tubular necrosis**
	  - ischemia
	  - toxins: aminoglycosides
	                iodinated contrast agents
	                cadmium
	                cisplatin
	
	2. acute glomerulonephritis
	3. acute pyelonephritis
	
	4. rhabdomyolysis (crash injury)

postrenal causes	**1. obstruction**
	  - stones
	  - strictures
	  - tumors

130

ASSESSMENT

◊ Nausea
◊ Headache, lethargy
• Edema
• Hypertension due to volume retention

LAB:

• Oliguria (<400 mL/day)
• Azotemia (=nitrogen retention: BUN > 20 mg/dL)
• Acidosis (pH < 7.35)

ANALYSIS

• Adequate urinary elimination?
• Fluid and electrolyte balance?
• Risk of cardiac arrhythmia due to hyperkalemia

IMPLEMENTATION

• Bed rest
• Monitor intake and output closely, weigh daily
• Monitor BUN and creatinine
• Watch for signs of hyperkalemia:
  - diarrhea
  - paresthesias
  - ECG changes
• Avoid: IV contrast studies
• Avoid: sulfonylureas and tetracyclines

DIET:

• High-carbohydrate
• Low-protein
• Low-sodium
• Low-potassium if hyperkalemia develops

7.8.) CHRONIC RENAL FAILURE

➤ **Most common causes:** hypertension, diabetes and glomerulonephritis

uremia	- increased BUN, increased creatinine - urine volume may be low or normal - anemia - bleeding tendency - encephalopathy
hypertriglyceridemia	- increased production of triglycerides - cholesterol levels normal - premature atherosclerosis
metabolic acidosis	- impaired NH_3 synthesis by kidneys limits H^+ excretion

Uremia = signs and symptoms of chronic renal failure
Azotemia = increased levels of nitrogenous compounds (<u>early</u> sign of uremia)

HEMODIALYSIS	PERITONEAL DIALYSIS
Client is attached to dialysis machine via a surgically created AV shunt	*Dialyzing fluid is introduced via catheter into peritoneal cavity*
4 hours, 3 times per week	4 exchanges a day, 7 days a week
<u>Complications of AV fistula</u>: - infection - thrombosis - ischemia of hand	<u>Complications</u>: - peritonitis - bleeding

ASSESSMENT

◊ Anorexia, nausea
◊ Lethargy
- Breath smells like ammonia
- Skin itching
- Edema
- Hypertension due to volume retention
- Confusion → apathy → coma

LAB:
- Anemia (lack of erythropoietin production by kidneys)
- Acidosis, hyperkalemia
- Uremia, azotemia

↓

ANALYSIS

- Adequate urinary elimination?
- Fluid and electrolyte balance?
- Altered thought process due to uremic toxins

↓

IMPLEMENTATION

- Monitor intake and output closely, weigh daily
- Watch for signs of pulmonary edema: dyspnea, rales
- Watch for signs of hyperkalemia:
  - diarrhea
  - paresthesia
  - ECG changes

↓

CLIENT EDUCATION

- Frequent nutritious meals, high in calories
- **low-protein, low-sodium, low-potassium diet**

Phosphate retention → bone demineralization (osteodystrophy)

133

7.9.) <u>KIDNEY TRANSPLANTATION</u>

<u>COMPLICATIONS</u>:
➤ Graft rejection
➤ Infections due to immunosuppression
➤ Recurrent disease

<u>SIGNS OF REJECTION</u>:
◊ Tenderness of transplant
• Fever
• Oliguria
• Hypertension
• Increasing serum creatinine

Organ donors wanted !

7.10.) <u>PROSTATE HYPERTROPHY</u>
Slow, benign enlargement of prostate – very common in elderly men!

ASSESSMENT
◊ Decreased force of urination (hesitancy)
◊ Nocturia
• Urinary retention → risk of infection
• Enlarged prostate on rectal exam

IMPLEMENTATION
• Monitor urine output and characteristics
• Encourage fluid intake
• Prepare client for prostate resection
MEDICATIONS:
• α-blockers (relaxes bladder sphincter, facilitates voiding)
• Finasteride (blocks conversion of testosterone to DHT)
POSTOPERATIVE:
• Kegel exercises
• Avoid straining and sex for 1-2 months

7.11.) <u>PROSTATE CANCER</u>

➢ Prostate carcinoma is the most common carcinoma in the male.
➢ Localized (curable) carcinoma in 60% of cases.
➢ Metastasizes to bones - back pain often first symptom of advanced disease.

ASSESSMENT

◊ Early tumor often asymptomatic!
  (teach client importance of regular rectal exams and check-ups)
◊ Back pain (from metastases)
• Urinary retention, dribbling
• Enlarged prostate on rectal exam
LAB:
• Elevated serum acid phosphatase
• Elevated PSA
• Elevated alkaline phosphatase indicates metastases to bones

---

IMPLEMENTATION

• Encourage patient to express fears
POSTOPERATIVE:
• Monitor drainage
• Monitor for signs of internal bleeding → shock
• Monitor for signs of infection

RADIOTHERAPY (for local disease):
• Expect nausea, vomiting, dry skin
ESTROGEN THERAPY (for metastatic disease):
• Expect gynecomastia, fluid retention

➢ **Transurethral resection:**   - Monitor for signs of urethral strictures
                                        (pain or straining to urinate)
➢ **Perineal resection:**   - Provide "Sitz baths" to relieve inflammation
➢ **Suprapubic resection:**   - Meticulous catheter care: keep skin clean and dry

SEXUALLY TRANSMITTED DISEASES

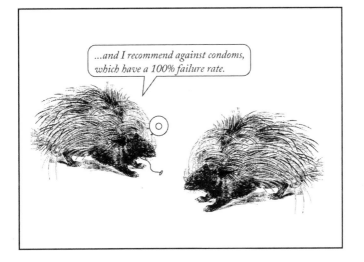

8.1.) SEXUALLY TRANSMITTED DISEASES

➢ Chlamydia is the most frequent STD in the US. May lead to infertility!
➢ Genital warts (papilloma virus) may lead to cervical cancer.
➢ Over 20 million people in US have genital herpes.
➢ Abstinence is the only 100% effective method to prevent HIV and STDs

	ORGANISM	SIGNS & SYMPTOMS
gonorrhea	*Gonococcus*	◊ **often asymptomatic** • or purulent discharge
NGU	*Chlamydia trachomatis*	◊ **often asymptomatic** • or urethritis/cervicitis
syphilis	*Treponema pallidum*	1°: **painless** ulcer (hard chancre) 2°: skin rash 3°: gumma or CNS involvement
chancroid	*Hemophilus ducreyi*	• **painful** ulcer (soft chancre)
genital herpes	*Herpes virus type 2* (sometimes type 1)	• **painful**, recurrent vesicles
genital warts	*Papilloma virus*	◊ **painless** • risk of cervical dysplasia and cancer

NGU = nongonococcal urethritis, often coexists with gonorrhea.

138

8.2.) AIDS

High risk groups:
- Homosexual or bisexual men and their partners
- Intravenous drug users
- Blood transfusion recipients before 1985
- Babies of mothers who are HIV positive

Clients are HIV infected if:
- HIV positive on ELISA blood test and confirmed by Western blot

Clients have AIDS if:
- HIV positive on ELISA blood test and confirmed by Western blot
- plus - CD4 lymphocytes < 200 cells/mm^3
  - or CD4 lymphocytes < 14%
  - or presence of opportunistic diseases

Acute Retroviral Syndrome
flu-like, occurs 2~4 weeks after infection

ASSESSMENT
- ◊ Myalgia
- Fever
- Lymphadenopathy
- Pharyngitis
- Rash

LAB:
- Thrombocytopenia
- Leukopenia
- HIV antigen not detectable by routine tests until 3-6 months after infection!

This can be fairly mild and non-specific. Many client's do not remember it.

8.3.) AIDS: SIGNS & SYMPTOMS

fever	- opportunistic **infections** - opportunistic **malignancies**
skin	- *Herpes zoster* - *Candida* - Kaposi sarcoma: purple/brown nodules, usually on toes and leg (more common in homosexual AIDS patients)
cough	- **BACTERIAL PNEUMONIA:** - ***Pneumocystis jirovecii* pneumonia** - **tuberculosis** (may be multi-drug-resistant)
dysphagia	- *Candida* - *Herpes simplex* - aphthous ulcers
diarrhea	- parasitic - bacterial (*Campylobacter, Salmonella, Shigella*)
headache	- bacterial meningitis - neurosyphilis - cryptococcosis - toxoplasmosis

In clients with exertional dyspnea and persistent dry cough
suspect **Pneumocystis jirovecii** *pneumonia*

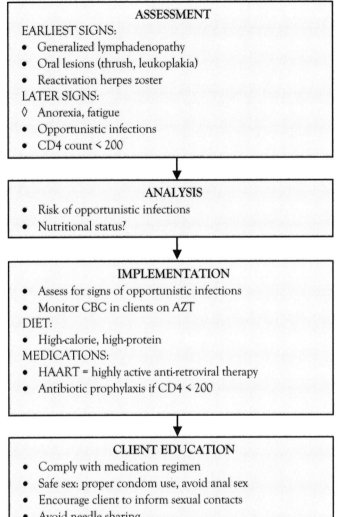

ASSESSMENT

EARLIEST SIGNS:
- Generalized lymphadenopathy
- Oral lesions (thrush, leukoplakia)
- Reactivation herpes zoster

LATER SIGNS:
◊ Anorexia, fatigue
- Opportunistic infections
- CD4 count < 200

ANALYSIS
- Risk of opportunistic infections
- Nutritional status?

IMPLEMENTATION
- Assess for signs of opportunistic infections
- Monitor CBC in clients on AZT

DIET:
- High-calorie, high-protein

MEDICATIONS:
- HAART = highly active anti-retroviral therapy
- Antibiotic prophylaxis if CD4 < 200

CLIENT EDUCATION
- Comply with medication regimen
- Safe sex: proper condom use, avoid anal sex
- Encourage client to inform sexual contacts
- Avoid needle sharing

HAART (multi-drug regimen):
➤ Decreases rate of maternal-fetal transmission
➤ Delays progression of HIV infection
➤ Significantly improves survival

 Never assume that family knows! Maintain confidentiality!

INFECTIOUS
DISEASES

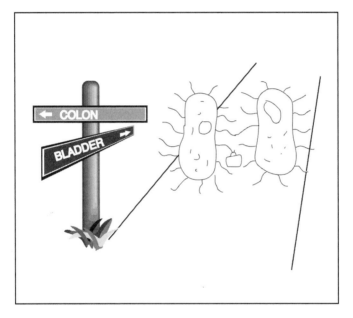

Marge and Phil leave the crowded city for
the less crowded suburbs.

9.1.) KEY LIST

CHARTS IN THIS BOOK WITH INFECTIOUS DISEASE INFO:

1.6	Universal Precautions	17.9	Pelvic Inflammatory Disease
4.19	Rheumatic Heart Disease	18.22	Puerperal Fever
4.22	Endocarditis	18.23	Mastitis
5.6	Upper Respiratory Infections	20.10	Neonatal Sepsis
5.7	Pneumonia	21.5	Infectious Diseases of
5.8	Tuberculosis		Childhood
5.10	Chronic Bronchitis	21.6	Incubation Periods
6.15	Hepatitis	21.8	Respiratory Tract Infections
7.3	Lower Urinary Tract Infections	21.9	Croup
8.1	Sexually Transmitted Diseases	21.10	Epiglottitis
8.2	AIDS	21.11	Otitis Media
12.11	Osteomyelitis	21.12	Tonsillitis
13.9	Meningitis	21.14	Rheumatic Fever
14.4	Conjunctivitis	23.3	Antibiotics

9.2.) SIGNS & SYMPTOMS

Kernig's sign	- **meningeal irritation** - patient supine, at first flex hip and knee - attempt to extend knee → pain or spasm occur
Brudzinski's sign	- **meningeal irritation** - patient supine, gently flex neck forward → flexion of hips and knees occur
opisthotonus	- **meningeal irritation** - severe muscle spasm causing back arch - more common in infants
McBurney's sign	- **appendicitis** - rebound tenderness at McBurney's point (1/3 from ant. sup. spine to umbilicus)
Murphy's sign	- **acute cholecystitis** - arrest of inspiration when palpating liver
Koplik's spots	- **measles** - small red spots with bluish-white center on buccal mucosa - generalized rash will follow in 1~2 days
Janeway spots	- **infective endocarditis** - tiny red lesions on palms and soles
Roth spots	- **infective endocarditis** - subretinal hemorrhages with pale center
Osler's nodes	- **infective endocarditis** - tender, raised nodules on finger pads and toes

Neisseria bacteria as seen under the microscope:

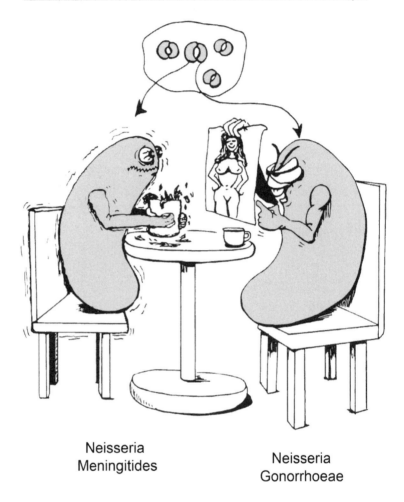

Neisseria
Meningitides

Neisseria
Gonorrhoeae

From Gladwin and Trattler: *Clinical Microbiology Made Ridiculously Simple*, MedMaster, 2008

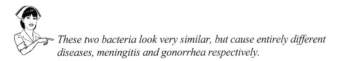

These two bacteria look very similar, but cause entirely different diseases, meningitis and gonorrhea respectively.

9.3.) DEFENSE MECHANISMS

	KEY FEATURES
skin barrier	- protects against staphylococci, streptococci etc.
IgM antibodies	- antibody response (first encounter)
IgG antibodies	- antibody response (subsequent encounter) - transferred via placenta to fetus!
IgA antibodies	- found in all mucous secretions - protect against colonizing flora
IgE antibodies	- on mast cells and basophils - mediate anaphylaxis and allergy
lymphocytes	- B cells produce antibodies - T cells regulate immune response (CD4 helper cells & CD8 suppressor cells) - "Natural killer cells" attack bacteria
neutrophils	- defective neutrophils → bacterial infections

9.4.) NOSOCOMIAL INFECTIONS

➤ 3~5% of hospital patients acquire a new infection during their stay!

➤ Sources of infection: visitors, other patients, personnel
➤ Inadequate hand washing of personnel
➤ Reservoirs: water tanks, air conditioning
➤ Invasive devices are a major risk factor

	RISK FACTORS
urinary tract infections	- duration of catheterization - absence of systemic antibiotics - more common in females
lower respiratory tract infections	- aspiration - decreased gag reflex
surgical wound infections	- duration of procedure - level of contamination - severity of illness **recommended antibiotic prophylaxis**: 2h before until 24h after operation
sepsis *mortality about 25%*	**primary** - intravenous cannulas **secondary** - urinary tract infections - pulmonary infections - cutaneous infections - wound infections

148

DISEASES
OF THE BLOOD

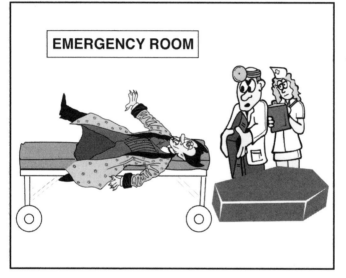

"Now how could he have A, B, AB, O, Rh- and Rh+
on the same type and cross match"?

10.1.) BLOOD

Serum = plasma minus fibrinogen

albumin	- provides osmotic pressure (low albumin → edema) - binds hormones, drugs ...
γ-globulin	- antibodies (=humoral immunity)

10.2.) BLOOD CELLS

	CAUSES
erythrocytosis	- lack of oxygen: high altitude, COPD
leukocytosis	- infections - leukemia
neutrophils: eosinophils: lymphocytes:	- infections, acute stress - allergies, parasites - viral infections, TBC
leukopenia	- radiation - bone marrow suppression
thrombocytopenia	- DIC - bone marrow suppression

10.3.) RED BLOOD CELLS

hematocrit	percentage of RBCs in blood volume
	- male adult: 40 ~ 50%
	- female adult: 35 ~ 45%

hemoglobin	oxygen carrying protein in red blood cells
	- male adult: 14~16 g/dL
	- female adult: 12~15 g/dL

Hematocrit may be false low if blood is obtained with capillary fingerstick ("milking").

direct Coombs' test	test for antibodies on patient's *erythrocytes*
positive if:	- hemolytic transfusion reaction (mismatch)
	- autoimmune hemolytic anemia
	- erythroblastosis fetalis [1]

indirect Coombs' test	test for antibodies in patient's *serum*
positive if:	- sensitization from previous transfusion
	- Rh sensitization from previous pregnancy

[1] *maternal antibodies bind to fetal RBCs → hemolysis*

10.4.) <u>ANEMIAS</u>

acute blood loss	- hematocrit remains normal in acute phase!
chronic blood loss	- may lead to iron deficiency
iron deficiency	- search for occult bleeding, especially in elderl
Vit. B12 or folic acid deficiency	- required for RBC maturation in bone marrow **Alcoholics:** B12 and folate deficiency common **Pregnancy:** Folate deficiency common: *give supplements!*
pernicious anemia	- chronic gastritis type A (autoimmune disease) - antibodies against intrinsic factor from stomac → reduced vit. B12 absorption in small bowel:
sickle cell anemia	- abnormal hemoglobin (electrophoresis) - "sickle cells" seen on blood smear - painful crises, leg ulcers
thalassemias	- abnormal hemoglobin (electrophoresis) - "target cells" on blood smear
hemolysis	- antibodies against RBCs - fragile RBCs

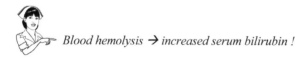

Blood hemolysis → increased serum bilirubin !

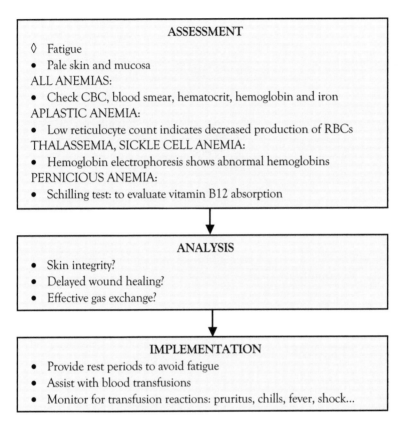

ASSESSMENT
◊ Fatigue
• Pale skin and mucosa
ALL ANEMIAS:
• Check CBC, blood smear, hematocrit, hemoglobin and iron
APLASTIC ANEMIA:
• Low reticulocyte count indicates decreased production of RBCs
THALASSEMIA, SICKLE CELL ANEMIA:
• Hemoglobin electrophoresis shows abnormal hemoglobins
PERNICIOUS ANEMIA:
• Schilling test: to evaluate vitamin B12 absorption

ANALYSIS
• Skin integrity?
• Delayed wound healing?
• Effective gas exchange?

IMPLEMENTATION
• Provide rest periods to avoid fatigue
• Assist with blood transfusions
• Monitor for transfusion reactions: pruritus, chills, fever, shock...

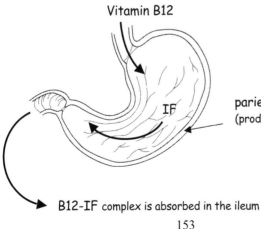

Vitamin B12

parietal cells
(produce intrinsic factor IF)

IF

B12-IF complex is absorbed in the ileum

10.5.) BLOOD PRODUCTS

	USED FOR:
whole blood	<u>active bleeding</u>, massive transfusions (packed RBC are preferred: less volume load)
fresh frozen plasma	bleeding patient with <u>coagulation deficiency</u>: - chronic liver disease - alcoholics - DIC
cryoprecipitate	DIC (to replace <u>fibrinogen</u>)
factor VIII or IX concentrate	hemophilia (to replace missing <u>factors</u>)

TRANSFUSION RISKS IN USA:

Febrile reaction	1 : 100
ABO incompatibility [1]	1 : 10,000
Hepatitis B	1 : 250,000
HIV or Hepatitis C	1 : 2,000,000

[1] *Most fatal transfusion reactions are due to a mismatch caused by clerical error !!!*

10.6.) <u>TRANSFUSION REACTIONS</u>

patients with this blood type:	have these serum antibodies:
O	A and B
A	B
B	A
AB	--
Rh negative	may or may not have Rh antibodies (only if previous contact with Rh+ blood)

ASSESSMENT

HEMOLYTIC REACTION (after 10-20 minutes):
◊ Chills, headache
◊ Lower back pain
• Flushing, "head feels full"
• Signs of shock
• Acute renal failure (oliguria)

FEBRILE REACTION (after 30 minutes):
◊ Chills, headache
• Elevated temperature

ALLERGIC REACTION:
• Pruritus
• Hives, wheezes
• Anaphylaxis

IMPLEMENTATION

HEMOLYTIC OR FEBRILE REACTION:
• Immediately stop transfusion
• Keep IV access – replace blood transfusion with normal saline
• Call physician

ALLERGIC REACTION:
• If hives are the only sign: proceed at slower rate (check institutional guidelines!)
• Prepare epinephrine if signs of anaphylaxis occur

Start infusion slowly (2 mL/min) to observe for early reaction. Stay at bedside.

10.7.) <u>ACUTE LEUKEMIA</u>

ALL (3~7 years) prognosis is fair	AML (all ages) prognosis is poor
◊ Fatigue, weakness, anorexia • Fever • Petechiae [1] • Ecchymoses [2]	◊ Fatigue, weakness, anorexia • Fever • Petechiae • Ecchymoses • Lymphadenopathy, splenomegaly • Auer rods in myeloblasts

[1] = *numerous tiny bruises (size of pinheads)*
[2] = *large-area bruises*

ANALYSIS
• Risk of injury and infections
• Effective coping?

↓

IMPLEMENTATION
• Monitor vital signs
• Watch for bleeding
• Watch for signs of infection
• Minimize side effects of chemotherapy

 Bleeding and infection are the major causes of death.

10.8.) CHRONIC LEUKEMIA

CML (50 years) prognosis is poor	**CLL (70 years)** prognosis is fair
◊ Fatigue, weakness, anorexia • Fever • Night sweats • Splenomegaly • Philadelphia chromosome	◊ Insidious onset ◊ Few symptoms • Low Ig levels • Infections

ANALYSIS
- Risk of injury and infections
- Effective coping?

↓

IMPLEMENTATION
- Monitor vital signs
- Watch for bleeding
- Watch for signs of infection
- Minimize side effects of chemotherapy

10.9.) <u>MULTIPLE MYELOMA</u>

Neoplasm of plasma cells - infiltrates bones, skull and vertebrae

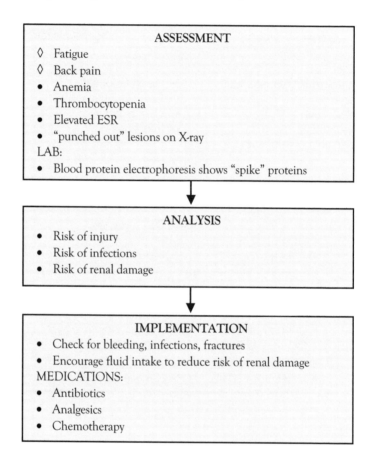

ASSESSMENT
- ◊ Fatigue
- ◊ Back pain
- • Anemia
- • Thrombocytopenia
- • Elevated ESR
- • "punched out" lesions on X-ray

LAB:
- • Blood protein electrophoresis shows "spike" proteins

ANALYSIS
- • Risk of injury
- • Risk of infections
- • Risk of renal damage

IMPLEMENTATION
- • Check for bleeding, infections, fractures
- • Encourage fluid intake to reduce risk of renal damage

MEDICATIONS:
- • Antibiotics
- • Analgesics
- • Chemotherapy

Abnormal immunoglobulins are produced by neoplastic plasma cells. These proteins can be filtered into the urine (=Bence Jones proteins) and severely damage the kidneys !

10.10.) LYMPHOMA

Neoplasm of lymph nodes

HODGKIN'S DISEASE	NON-HODGKIN LYMPHOMAS
- no leukemic component - spreads from lymph node to lymph node	- often have leukemic component - common in AIDS patients

ASSESSMENT
◊ Weakness, fatigue
◊ Loss of appetite
◊ Fever, night sweats
• Painless enlargement of lymph nodes
• Enlarged liver and spleen
• Diagnosis: Lymph node biopsy

ANALYSIS
• Risk of injury
• Risk of infections

IMPLEMENTATION
• Monitor for signs of infection
• Provide comfort measures for fever and night sweats
CHEMOTHERAPY:
• For generalized disease
• ABVD, CHOP or some other drug combination
RADIOTHERAPY:
• For localized disease
• Skin care: water, mild soaps. Avoid rubbing.

Immediately report fever or any other sign of infection !

10.11.) <u>BLEEDING DISORDERS</u>

platelet defect	- bleeding into **skin and mucous membranes** - males and females
coagulation defect	- bleeding into **joints, muscle, viscera** - mainly males
vascular defect	- **purpura** [1] - gastrointestinal bleeding - mainly females

[1] *bleeding into skin*

Prolonged use of a tourniquet before drawing blood sample may falsely increase PTT and PT !

10.12.) THROMBOCYTOPENIA

> Platelets < 100,000/µL increased bleeding risk
> Platelets < 20,000/µL spontaneous bleeding
> Platelets < 10,000/µL CNS bleeding

	CAUSES
bone marrow failure	- viral infections - drugs - radiation
platelet destruction	- ITP
platelet consumption	- TTP - DIC
platelet sequestration	- splenomegaly

ASSESSMENT
◊　History of drugs/medication intake
◊　Fatigue
•　Easy bruising: petechiae, ecchymoses
•　Bleeding from mucosal surfaces

IMPLEMENTATION
•　Prevent avoidable injury
•　Avoid invasive procedures if possible
•　Apply pressure to venipuncture site until bleeding stops

CLIENT EDUCATION
•　Avoid aspirin (suppresses platelet activity)
•　Avoid coughing and straining
　　(increased blood pressure increases risk of CNS bleeding)

10.13.) <u>HEMOPHILIA</u>

hemophilia A	- **factor VIII deficiency** - X-linked recessive
hemophilia B	- **factor IX deficiency** - X-linked recessive
von Willebrand's	- **deficiency of von Willebrand Factor** - autosomal recessive or dominant

---

ASSESSMENT
- Excessive bruising
- Prolonged bleeding after minor injuries
- Nosebleeds
- Hemarthrosis (bleeding into joints: elbows, knees, ankles)

↓

IMPLEMENTATION
- When bleeding: Elevate and apply pressure for 10-20 min.
- Avoid taking rectal temperatures
- Treat hemarthroses early to preserve mobility of joint
  (elevation, ice packs, may require splinting)

MEDICATIONS:
- Replace coagulation factors VIII or IX with <u>recombinant</u> !
  (heat-treated only if recombinant factors are not available)

↓

CLIENT EDUCATION
- Avoid trauma whenever possible
- Never use aspirin (inhibits platelets and worsens bleeding)!
-

GENETIC COUNSELING:
- X-linked recessive disease: - transmitted by asymptomatic female carriers
  - 50% of male offspring will have disease
  - 50% of female offspring are carriers

10.14.) DIC
Disseminated Intravascular Coagulation

 Intravascular activation of coagulation causes consumption of coagulation factors. This results in thrombosis or bleeding tendency or both and is a very serious condition.

CAUSES OF DIC:
➢ Gram negative sepsis
➢ Adenocarcinomas
➢ Crash injury
➢ Amniotic fluid embolism

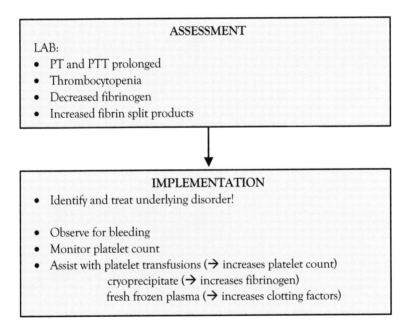

ASSESSMENT

LAB:
- PT and PTT prolonged
- Thrombocytopenia
- Decreased fibrinogen
- Increased fibrin split products

IMPLEMENTATION
- Identify and treat underlying disorder!

- Observe for bleeding
- Monitor platelet count
- Assist with platelet transfusions (➔ increases platelet count)
   cryoprecipitate (➔ increases fibrinogen)
   fresh frozen plasma (➔ increases clotting factors)

ENDOCRINE
DISEASES

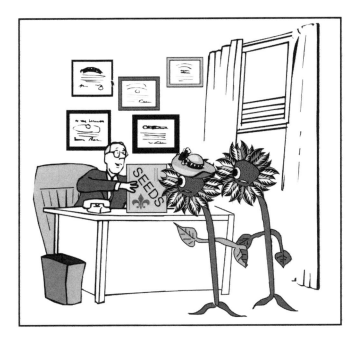

"Even though you can't have children of your own, there are other options. Try planting some of these."

11.1.) PHYSIOLOGY

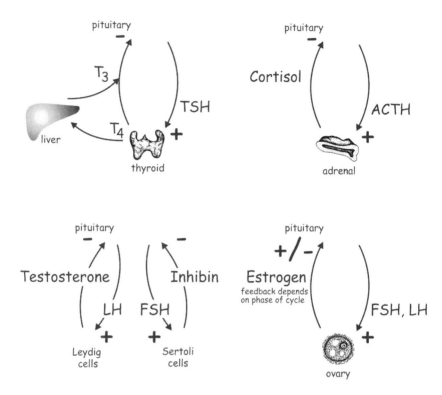

GONADOTROPE HORMONES:

	OVARIES	TESTES
FSH	follicle maturation	spermatogenesis
LH	triggers ovulation luteinization of follicle	testosterone secretion (Leydig cells)

HORMONE	SOURCE	FUNCTION
ADH	pituitary	conservation of water by kidneys
prolactin	pituitary	milk production during pregnancy
T3	thyroid	increases metabolism and heat production infants: stimulates growth and development
PTH	parathyroid	increases serum Ca^{2+} levels
aldosterone	adrenal	promotes resorption of Na^+ by kidneys promotes excretion of K^+ by kidneys
cortisol	adrenal	"stress" hormone highest level in morning hours increases blood sugar anti-inflammatory at high concentrations
insulin	pancreas	promotes sugar uptake and metabolism
testosterone	testes	sexual development secondary sexual characteristics of male [1] sperm production libido (sexual desire)
estrogen	ovaries	secondary sexual characteristics of female [2] follicle maturation (ovaries) thins cervical mucus
progesterone	ovaries	prepares and supports endometrium for pregnancy ("secretory change")

[1] *testes enlarge, axillary and pubic hair*   [2] *breasts enlarge*

11.2.) <u>PITUITARY HYPOFUNCTION</u>

LACK OF:	RESULTS IN:
FSH and LH ↓	**decreased sex hormones** • irregular menstruation • amenorrhea
ACTH ↓	**decreased cortisol** ◊ weakness ◊ malaise • nausea, vomiting
TSH ↓	**decreased thyroid hormones** ◊ depression ◊ apathy

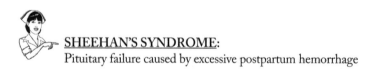

<u>SHEEHAN'S SYNDROME</u>:
Pituitary failure caused by excessive postpartum hemorrhage

11.3.) PITUITARY HYPERFUNCTION

Usually caused by pituitary adenomas

EXCESSIVE:	RESULTS IN:
prolactin ↑	**women** • galactorrhea • amenorrhea **men** ◊ loss of sexual desire • impotence • galactorrhea
GH ↑	**children** • giantism **adults** • acromegaly [1]
ACTH ↑	• signs of excess glucocorticoids • signs of excess mineralocorticoids

[1] *enlarged jaw, forehead, hands and feet*

11.4.) ACROMEGALY

Excessive GH in adults (due to pituitary adenoma)

ASSESSMENT

◊ Visual disturbance: hemianopia
(due to pressure of adenoma against optic nerve or tract)
- Growth of hands → increasing glove/ring size
- Growth of feet → increasing shoe size
- Growth of jaw → protruding lower jaw
- Increased blood sugar levels

DIAGNOSIS:
- Measurement of serum GH
- CT scan of head: enlarged sella turcica

IMPLEMENTATION
- Provide emotional support to help patient cope with altered body image
- Check for signs of diabetes: polyuria, polydipsia
- Prepare client for pituitary surgery

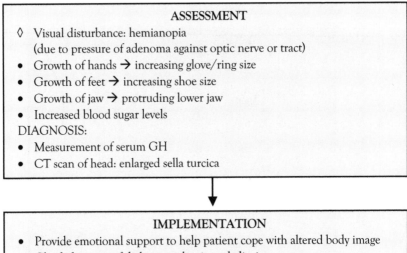

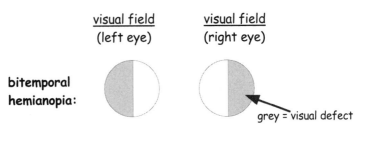

visual field (left eye)   visual field (right eye)

bitemporal hemianopia:

grey = visual defect

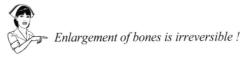

Enlargement of bones is irreversible !

11.5.) <u>CUSHING'S DISEASE</u>

Cushing's disease: pituitary adenoma → excessive ACTH → increased cortisol
Cushing's syndrome: adrenal adenoma → excessive cortisol → decreased ACTH

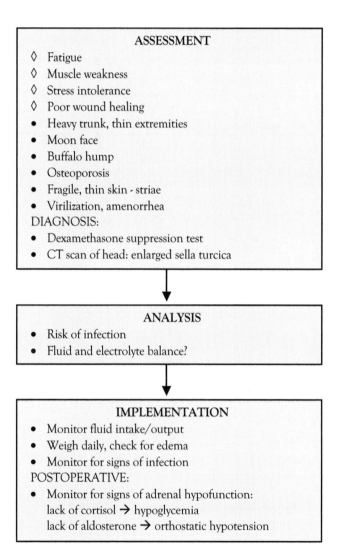

ASSESSMENT
◊ Fatigue
◊ Muscle weakness
◊ Stress intolerance
◊ Poor wound healing
• Heavy trunk, thin extremities
• Moon face
• Buffalo hump
• Osteoporosis
• Fragile, thin skin - striae
• Virilization, amenorrhea
DIAGNOSIS:
• Dexamethasone suppression test
• CT scan of head: enlarged sella turcica

ANALYSIS
• Risk of infection
• Fluid and electrolyte balance?

IMPLEMENTATION
• Monitor fluid intake/output
• Weigh daily, check for edema
• Monitor for signs of infection
POSTOPERATIVE:
• Monitor for signs of adrenal hypofunction:
  lack of cortisol → hypoglycemia
  lack of aldosterone → orthostatic hypotension

11.6.) CONN'S SYNDROME

Primary hyperaldosteronism (usually due to adrenal adenoma)

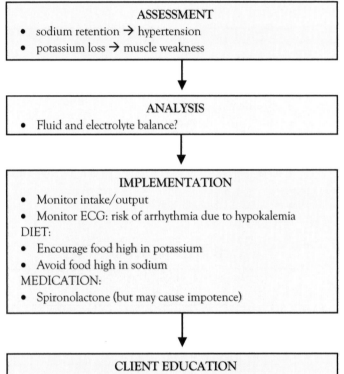

ASSESSMENT
- sodium retention → hypertension
- potassium loss → muscle weakness

ANALYSIS
- Fluid and electrolyte balance?

IMPLEMENTATION
- Monitor intake/output
- Monitor ECG: risk of arrhythmia due to hypokalemia

DIET:
- Encourage food high in potassium
- Avoid food high in sodium

MEDICATION:
- Spironolactone (but may cause impotence)

CLIENT EDUCATION
- Clients with <u>bilateral</u> adrenalectomy require lifelong replacement of gluco- and mineralocorticoids
- Take steroids with milk or antacids
- Carry medical identification card

<u>Hyperaldosteronism may also be secondary to:</u>
➤ Congestive heart failure
➤ Liver cirrhosis
➤ Nephrotic syndrome

11.7.) <u>ADDISON'S DISEASE</u>
Adrenal hypofunction (usually due to autoimmune disease)

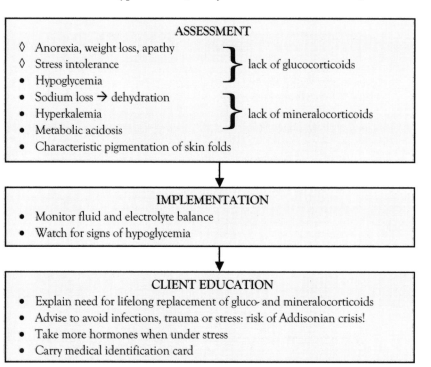

ASSESSMENT
◊ Anorexia, weight loss, apathy
◊ Stress intolerance   } lack of glucocorticoids
• Hypoglycemia
• Sodium loss → dehydration
• Hyperkalemia   } lack of mineralocorticoids
• Metabolic acidosis
• Characteristic pigmentation of skin folds

IMPLEMENTATION
• Monitor fluid and electrolyte balance
• Watch for signs of hypoglycemia

CLIENT EDUCATION
• Explain need for lifelong replacement of gluco- and mineralocorticoids
• Advise to avoid infections, trauma or stress: risk of Addisonian crisis!
• Take more hormones when under stress
• Carry medical identification card

11.8.) <u>ADDISONIAN CRISIS</u>
Lack of glucocorticoids → minor stress or illness may cause fatal crisis

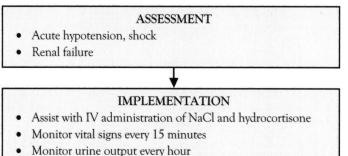

ASSESSMENT
• Acute hypotension, shock
• Renal failure

IMPLEMENTATION
• Assist with IV administration of NaCl and hydrocortisone
• Monitor vital signs every 15 minutes
• Monitor urine output every hour

11.9.) HYPERTHYROIDISM

Graves' disease: antibodies to TSH receptors stimulate thyroid

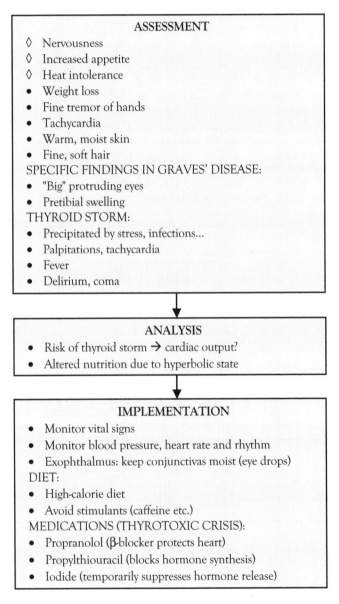

ASSESSMENT
◊ Nervousness
◊ Increased appetite
◊ Heat intolerance
• Weight loss
• Fine tremor of hands
• Tachycardia
• Warm, moist skin
• Fine, soft hair

SPECIFIC FINDINGS IN GRAVES' DISEASE:
• "Big" protruding eyes
• Pretibial swelling

THYROID STORM:
• Precipitated by stress, infections...
• Palpitations, tachycardia
• Fever
• Delirium, coma

ANALYSIS
• Risk of thyroid storm → cardiac output?
• Altered nutrition due to hyperbolic state

IMPLEMENTATION
• Monitor vital signs
• Monitor blood pressure, heart rate and rhythm
• Exophthalmus: keep conjunctivas moist (eye drops)

DIET:
• High-calorie diet
• Avoid stimulants (caffeine etc.)

MEDICATIONS (THYROTOXIC CRISIS):
• Propranolol (β-blocker protects heart)
• Propylthiouracil (blocks hormone synthesis)
• Iodide (temporarily suppresses hormone release)

11.10.) <u>HYPOTHYROIDISM</u>
(Myxedema)

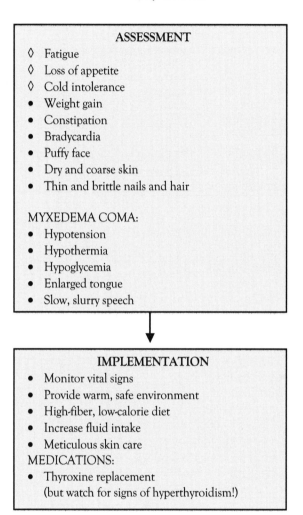

ASSESSMENT
◊ Fatigue
◊ Loss of appetite
◊ Cold intolerance
• Weight gain
• Constipation
• Bradycardia
• Puffy face
• Dry and coarse skin
• Thin and brittle nails and hair

MYXEDEMA COMA:
• Hypotension
• Hypothermia
• Hypoglycemia
• Enlarged tongue
• Slow, slurry speech

IMPLEMENTATION
• Monitor vital signs
• Provide warm, safe environment
• High-fiber, low-calorie diet
• Increase fluid intake
• Meticulous skin care
MEDICATIONS:
• Thyroxine replacement
  (but watch for signs of hyperthyroidism!)

11.11.) DIABETES MELLITUS

➢ IDDM:
Pancreas does not produce insulin (destruction of islet cells)
➢ NIDDM:
Pancreas produces insulin but patient's cells are resistant to insulin

	IDDM	NIDDM
onset	juvenile	adult
body weight	normal	obese
ketoacidosis	common	rare

➢ *Normal glucose levels: 60 –100 mg/dL (blood) or 70–110 mg/dL (serum).*

KETOACIDOSIS	HYPOGLYCEMIC COMA
◊ Nausea, vomiting ◊ Drowsiness • Acetone breath • Dehydration • Kussmaul respiration LAB: • Increased serum glucose • Increased serum osmolarity • Serum pH < 7.4	◊ Confusion, weakness ◊ Anxiety, irritability • Pallor • Tachycardia • Sweating • Seizures • Coma

Ketoacidosis is often precipitated by infections, stress or trauma.
Hypoglycemia is often precipitated by unusual physical exercise by clients on insulin.

ASSESSMENT

◊ Fatigue
◊ Polydipsia
◊ Polyuria, nocturia
• Elevated fasting glucose
• IDDM: Weight loss
• NIDDM: Weight gain
• Glucosuria (dipstick+ if plasma glucose > 180 mg/dL)

IMPLEMENTATION

• Monitor intake/output
• Monitor serum glucose, urine glucose
• Monitor for signs of insulin shock (hypoglycemia)
• Assess for diabetic neuropathy:
    decreased sensation → increased risk of injury!
• Watch for foot wounds or blisters!
DIET:
• **NIDDM:** Weight loss may reverse diabetes
• **IDDM:** Regular meal times and caloric content
KETOACIDOSIS:
• Assist with IV fluids, electrolytes and insulin
• Potassium replacement
• Monitor vital signs
• Monitor intake/output hourly

CLIENT EDUCATION

• Teach importance of home glucose monitoring to reduce risk of long-term complications (accelerated arteriosclerosis):

DIABETIC COMPLICATIONS:

➢ Coronary artery disease → MI (often "silent")
➢ Cerebrovascular disease → stroke
➢ Foot ischemia → gangrene
➢ Retinopathy → blindness
➢ Nephropathy → renal failure

177

11.12.) <u>INSULIN</u>
for treatment of IDDM

➢ Insulin is measured in units.
  Most common is U-100 insulin (containing 100 U/mL)

		PEAK	**DURATION**
"regular"	fast acting	30 min	120 min
NPH	intermediate acting	8-12 h	18-24 h
PZI	long acting	24 h	36 h

<u>EXAMPLE</u>:
Doctor's order: Humulin Regular 10 U s.c. and Humulin NPH 25 U s.c. a.c.

Draw up 0.1 cc regular, then draw up 0.25 cc NPH insulin, and give subcutaneously before meal.

When mixing two types of insulin in same syringe: Always draw up regular first!

<u>RISKS & SIDE-EFFECTS</u>:
➢ Hypoglycemic reactions: sweating, anxiety, tremor, weakness
➢ Risk of allergy: beef > pork > human insulin
➢ Fat atrophy at site of injection

11.13.) <u>SULFONYLUREAS</u>
for treatment of NIDDM

➢ Sulfonylureas should not be given to patients with liver or kidney failure: Accumulation of drug will increase risk of hypoglycemia.

	DURATION
tolbutamide	8 h
glyburide, glipizide	20 h, most potent
chlorpropamide	48 h

Advise clients to take medication in morning to avoid hypoglycemic reaction at night!

11.14.) <u>METABOLIC SYNDROME</u>

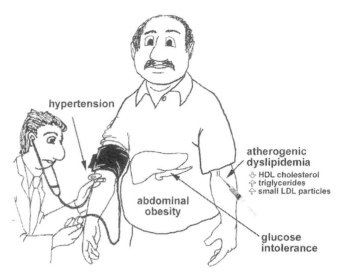

From Chizner: *Clinical Cardiology Made Ridiculously Simple*, MedMaster, 2010

<u>METABOLIC SYNDROME - if at least three of these are present</u>:

- Waist circumference >40 inches (men) or >35 inches (women)
- Triglycerides >150 mg/dL
- HDL cholesterol <40mg/dL (men) or <50 mg/dL (women)
- Blood pressure >130/85 mmHg
- Fasting glucose >100 mg/dL

Patients with metabolic syndrome are at increased risk of coronary heart disease and diseases related to plaque buildups in artery walls and also type-2 diabetes. Probably over 50 million Americans have this!

MUSCULOSKELETAL
DISEASES

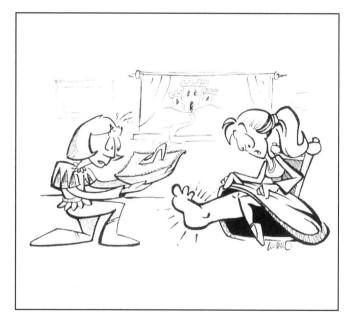

Cinderella's untimely episode of pedal edema

12.1.) <u>SIGNS & SYMPTOMS</u>

Heberden's nodes	- **osteoarthritis** - painless bony enlargement of DIP
swan neck deformity	- **rheumatoid arthritis** - hyperextended PIP - slightly flexed DIP also: - volar subluxation of MCP - ulnar deviation of fingers
tophi	- **gout** - painless, nodular swelling (uric acid deposits) - ears, hands, feet

PIP = *proximal interphalangeal joint*
DIP = *distal interphalangeal joint*
MCP = *metacarpophalangeal joint*

12.2.) <u>ASSESSMENT: ARTHRITIS</u>

RHEUMATOID ARTHRITIS	OSTEOARTHRITIS
autoimmune disease	**degenerative disease**

◊ Morning stiffness
• Swelling of 3 or more joints
• Involves: wrist, MCP and PIP
 	
• Subcutaneous nodules
• Rheumatoid factor in serum
• <u>Characteristic hand deformity</u>:
  - ulnar deviation of digits
  - "swan neck" deformity
 	
X-ray:
• Joint erosions
• Periarticular bone erosions
	◊ Progressive pain
	◊ Relieved by rest
	• Involves weight bearing joints
	  - hip joint, knee joint
	  (- also DIP and PIP in women)
	
	X-ray:
	• Loss of cartilage
	• Narrowed joint space
	• Subchondral cysts and sclerosis
	• New bone formation
	  (marginal osteophytes)

<u>Ulnar deviation</u>:

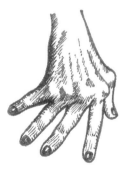

<u>Swan neck deformity</u>:

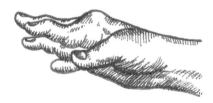

12.3.) <u>OSTEOARTHRITIS</u>

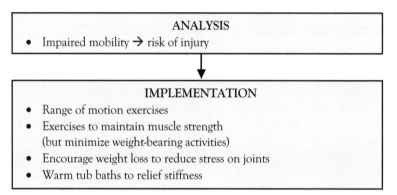

ANALYSIS
- Impaired mobility → risk of injury

IMPLEMENTATION
- Range of motion exercises
- Exercises to maintain muscle strength
  (but minimize weight-bearing activities)
- Encourage weight loss to reduce stress on joints
- Warm tub baths to relief stiffness

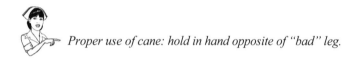

Proper use of cane: hold in hand opposite of "bad" leg.

12.4.) <u>RHEUMATOID ARTHRITIS</u>

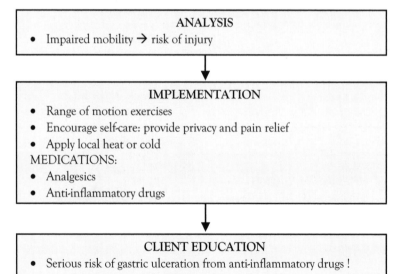

ANALYSIS
- Impaired mobility → risk of injury

IMPLEMENTATION
- Range of motion exercises
- Encourage self-care: provide privacy and pain relief
- Apply local heat or cold
MEDICATIONS:
- Analgesics
- Anti-inflammatory drugs

CLIENT EDUCATION
- Serious risk of gastric ulceration from anti-inflammatory drugs !

12.5.) GOUT

Deposits of urate crystals in synovial tissue → acute inflammation

---

ASSESSMENT
◊ May be asymptomatic for a long time
◊ Acute attack: pain in joint of great toe (called "podagra")
• Elevated serum uric acid
• Tophi: urate deposits in subcutaneous tissue

IMPLEMENTATION
• Bed rest during acute attack
• Use cradle to keep bedcovers elevated
• Encourage fluid intake (3L/day)
• Hot packs (reduce muscle spasm and pain)
• Cold packs (reduce swelling and pain)
MEDICATIONS:
• **Asymptomatic hyperuricemia:** no medication necessary
• **Mild attacks:** analgesics (acetaminophen)
• **Severe attacks:** colchicine, NSAIDs
• Allopurinol: reduces uric acid production
• Probenecid: increases renal uric acid excretion

CLIENT EDUCATION
• Encourage weight loss but avoid crash diets!
• Avoid alcohol
• Limit food high in purines (organ meat, anchovies, shellfish)

Factors that inhibit uric acid secretion:
(=increased risk of gout)
➢ Alcohol
➢ Aspirin
➢ Diuretcis

12.6.) SPONDYLOARTHROPATHIES
Autoimmune diseases involving spine and sacroiliac joint

ankylosing spondylitis	(more common in young men) ◊ gradual onset • **always sacroiliitis**

Reiter's syndrome
(reactive arthritis)
	(more common in men)
	
	◊ sudden onset
	• **urethritis**
	• **arthritis (knees, ankle)**
	
	  - follows dysentery (*Shigella*)
	  - follows STD (*Chlamydia*)

psoriatic arthritis	(more common in women) ◊ variable onset • occurs in 20% of psoriatic patients • nail pitting • "sausage toes"

Physical therapy, postural and breathing exercises are extremely important to maintain mobility and posture !

186

12.7.) <u>SYSTEMIC LUPUS ERYTHEMATOSUS</u>
Chronic inflammatory disease of connective tissues (autoimmune)

systemic lupus

◊ weakness, fatigue
◊ anorexia, weight loss
◊ photosensitivity
- **butterfly rash (spares nasolabial fold)**
- **discoid rash**
- anemia
- arthritis
- nephrotic syndrome

LAB:
- leukopenia, lymphopenia
- thrombocytopenia
- antinuclear antibodies
- false positive tests for syphilis

---

drug induced lupus

◊ often fairly mild
◊ history of hydralazine or procainamide
- reversible after drug cessation

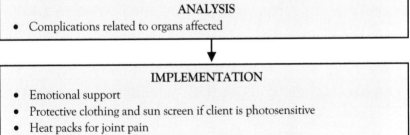

ANALYSIS
- Complications related to organs affected

↓

IMPLEMENTATION
- Emotional support
- Protective clothing and sun screen if client is photosensitive
- Heat packs for joint pain
- Monitor for signs of renal damage: edema, hypertension

MEDICATIONS:
- Steroids (topical for skin, systemic if organ involvement)

12.8.) <u>OSTEOPOROSIS</u>

Loss of bone mass → risk of fractures

➢ All elderly persons are at risk!
➢ Bone loss is accelerated in postmenopausal women (lack of estrogen)

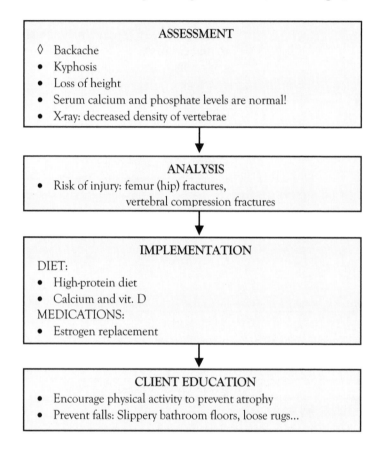

ASSESSMENT

◊ Backache
• Kyphosis
• Loss of height
• Serum calcium and phosphate levels are normal!
• X-ray: decreased density of vertebrae

ANALYSIS

• Risk of injury: femur (hip) fractures,
vertebral compression fractures

IMPLEMENTATION

DIET:
• High-protein diet
• Calcium and vit. D
MEDICATIONS:
• Estrogen replacement

CLIENT EDUCATION

• Encourage physical activity to prevent atrophy
• Prevent falls: Slippery bathroom floors, loose rugs...

Estrogens slightly <u>increase the risk</u> of endometrial cancer and breast cancer. Regular check-ups for clients on estrogen replacement are recommended.

12.9.) <u>HERNIATED DISK</u>

ASSESSMENT
◊ Severe lower back pain
◊ Pain radiating down buttocks and legs
◊ Usually unilateral
• Neurological exam: motor or sensory deficits are a
                very serious sign!
• Diagnosis: CT or MRI

ANALYSIS
• Risk of injury to spinal cord and nerve roots
• Level of mobility?

IMPLEMENTATION
• Apply local heat or cold
CERVICAL:
• Cervical herniation: Collar or traction required
LUMBAR:
• Bed rest until inflammation is reduced
• Provide firm mattress
• Recommend high-fiber diet with plenty of fluid
  (to prevent constipation and straining)

CLIENT EDUCATION
• Avoid prolonged sitting
• Use legs when lifting objects (keep spine straight)
• Exercise to strengthen abdominal and back muscles

12.10.) <u>CARPAL TUNNEL SYNDROME</u>

Compression of median nerve at wrist joint

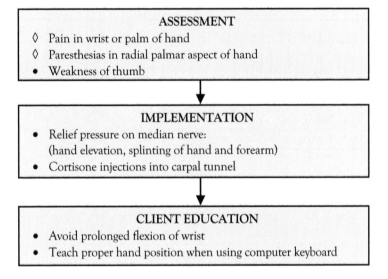

ASSESSMENT
◊ Pain in wrist or palm of hand
◊ Paresthesias in radial palmar aspect of hand
• Weakness of thumb

IMPLEMENTATION
• Relief pressure on median nerve:
  (hand elevation, splinting of hand and forearm)
• Cortisone injections into carpal tunnel

CLIENT EDUCATION
• Avoid prolonged flexion of wrist
• Teach proper hand position when using computer keyboard

A   B

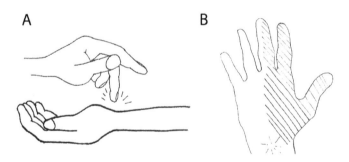

From Tétreault &Ouellette: *Orthopedics Made Ridiculously Simple*, MedMaster, 2009

Tinel Sign: Tapping on the wrist of the patient (A) triggers tingling and numbness in the median nerve territory (B, palmar view).

12.11.) <u>OSTEOMYELITIS</u>

Infection of bone, usually by *Staphylococcus aureus*

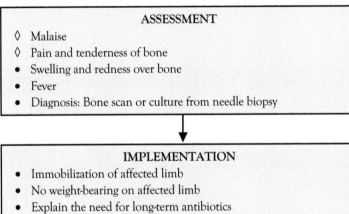

ASSESSMENT
◊ Malaise
◊ Pain and tenderness of bone
• Swelling and redness over bone
• Fever
• Diagnosis: Bone scan or culture from needle biopsy

IMPLEMENTATION
• Immobilization of affected limb
• No weight-bearing on affected limb
• Explain the need for long-term antibiotics
  (oral until 6 weeks after fever normalizes)

12.12.) LEG AMPUTATION

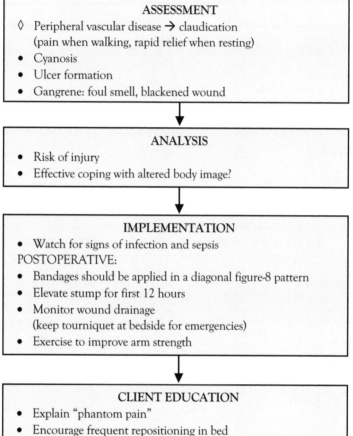

ASSESSMENT
◊ Peripheral vascular disease → claudication
  (pain when walking, rapid relief when resting)
- Cyanosis
- Ulcer formation
- Gangrene: foul smell, blackened wound

ANALYSIS
- Risk of injury
- Effective coping with altered body image?

IMPLEMENTATION
- Watch for signs of infection and sepsis
POSTOPERATIVE:
- Bandages should be applied in a diagonal figure-8 pattern
- Elevate stump for first 12 hours
- Monitor wound drainage
  (keep tourniquet at bedside for emergencies)
- Exercise to improve arm strength

CLIENT EDUCATION
- Explain "phantom pain"
- Encourage frequent repositioning in bed
- Massage stump to improve vascularity

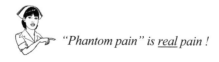

"Phantom pain" is <u>real</u> pain !

12.13.) <u>CRUTCHES & CANES</u>

<u>CRUTCHES</u>:

fitting	- measure from anterior fold of axilla to heel, add 6 inches - there should be 2 inch space between axillary fold and underarm piece to prevent damage to brachial plexus ("crutch paralysis")
basic stance	- crutches should rest in front and lateral of feet
2-point gait	1. advance right crutch and left foot together 2. advance left crutch and right foot together
3-point gait	***used if only one leg is injured*** 1. advance both crutches and involved leg forward 2. advance healthy foot while keeping body weight on crutches
4-point gait	***similar to 2-point gait, but slower and more stable*** 1. advance right crutch 2. advance left foot 3. advance left crutch 4. advance right foot

<u>CANES</u>:

fitting	- highest point should be at level of greater trochanter - hand piece should allow 30° flexion at elbow
use	- hold cane in hand opposite to injured leg - advance cane and injured leg at same time - don't lean body over cane

Walking upstairs: "good" leg first - walking downstairs: "bad" leg first !

DISEASES
OF THE
NERVOUS SYSTEM

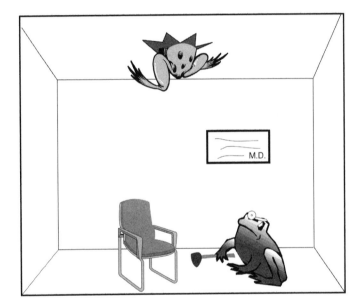

Hazards of amphibian neurology

13.1.) <u>SIGNS & SYMPTOMS</u>

decorticate posture	**legs extended, arms flexed** - damage above mid brain
decerebrate posture	**legs and arms extended, wrist pronation** - damage to mid brain
asterixis	**"flapping tremor"** (wrist joint and fingers) - liver failure
ataxia	**reeling, wide gait** - cerebellar disease - alcoholism
athetosis	**slow involuntary snakelike movements** (especially face, neck and upper extremities) - damage to basal ganglia
chorea	**bursts of rapid, jerky movements** - Huntington's disease (chorea plus intellectual decline) - rheumatic fever
cogwheel rigidity	**jerking of arm muscles when passively stretched** - cardinal sign of Parkinson's disease - side-effect of antipsychotic drugs
Gower's sign	**proximal muscle weakness** - characteristic way to rise from the floor (Duchenne's muscle atrophy)

13.2.) <u>GLASGOW COMA SCALE</u>

(coma = 7 points or less)

eye opening response	**1 point:** no response **2 points:** to pain **3 points:** to speech **4 points:** spontaneously
motor response	**1 point:** no response to pain **2 points:** abnormal extension (decerebrate) **3 points:** abnormal flexion (decorticate) **4 points:** withdraws from pain **5 points:** localizes pain **6 points:** obeys verbal commands
verbal response	**1 point:** no response **2 points:** incomprehensible sounds **3 points:** inappropriate words **4 points:** confused **5 points:** oriented to time, place and person

THE COMATOSE CLIENT:

> **ANALYSIS**
> - Effective breathing pattern?
> - Effective gas exchange?
> - Effective cardiac output?

> **IMPLEMENTATION**
> - Maintain open airways
> - Monitor vital signs frequently
> - Monitor neurological status frequently
> - Skin care: turn client frequently

13.3.) <u>CENTRAL NERVOUS SYSTEM</u>

	MAJOR FUNCTIONS	
frontal lobe	behavioral functions learned motor function language motor center	
parietal lobe	integrates sensory information spatial awareness	
temporal lobe	memory emotions language recognition	
occipital lobe	visual recognition	
basal ganglia	involuntary components of movement	
cerebellum	balance "fine-tuning" of movement	
brain stem	vital centers (respiration, cardiovascular)	

*The **dominant hemisphere** contains the language centers and is (in right-handed persons) usually the left brain.*

13.4.) AUTONOMIC NERVOUS SYSTEM

	SYMPATHETIC	PARASYMPATHETIC
heart	increased heart rate increased conduction increased force	decreased heart rate
bronchi	dilation	constriction
GI tract	reduced motility	increased motility
rectum	allows filling	empties rectum relaxes internal sphincter
bladder	allows filling	empties bladder relaxes internal sphincter
erection		maintains erection
ejaculation	triggers ejaculation	
pupils of eye	big (mydriasis)	small (miosis)
salivary glands		secretion
blood vessels	depends on receptors [1]: - α constricts - β dilates	

[1] *Examples:* - **Skin vessels have α receptors**
(clients in shock have pale skin)

- **Coronary arteries have β receptors**
(increased blood flow to heart during exercise)

13.5.) CRANIAL NERVES

		MAJOR FUNCTIONS
I.	Olfactory	smell
II.	Optic	vision
III. IV. VI.	Oculomotor Trochlear Abducent	eye movements
V.	Trigeminal	facial sensation jaw movements
VII.	Facial	taste facial expression
VIII.	Acoustic	hearing & balance
IX.	Glossopharyngeal	taste throat sensation gag and swallow
X.	Vagus	gag and swallow parasympathetic activity
XI.	Accessory	neck and back muscles
XII.	Hypoglossal	tongue movements

13.6.) <u>SLEEP DISORDERS</u>

➢ Discourage use of benzodiazepines (risk of dependence).
➢ Sleeping pills should be used for very short-term help only.

insomnia	◊ difficulty initiating sleep ◊ difficulty maintaining sleep • exclude medical conditions • exclude mental disorders such as anxiety or major depressive disorder
hypersomnia	◊ prolonged sleep ◊ daytime sleep • exclude insomnia, medical and mental conditions
narcolepsy	• REM onset sleep • cataplexy: sudden loss of muscle tone • sleep paralysis (very frightening experience: client awakes and finds himself unable to move for several minutes)
respiratory	• obstructive sleep apnea • central sleep apnea

__Teach client proper sleep hygiene:__
1. Keep regular bed times.
2. Use bedroom for sleeping only (don't read in bed).
3. Increase physical exercise during day.

13.7.) <u>HEADACHE</u>

tension headache	◊ **steady, nonpulsatile** ◊ unilateral or bilateral
classic migraine	◊ **preceded by aura** ◊ malaise ◊ nausea ◊ photophobia
common migraine	◊ **not preceded by aura** ◊ malaise ◊ nausea ◊ photophobia
tumor headache	◊ **develops slowly with increased** **intracranial pressure** ◊ initially mild, occurs after waking up ◊ exacerbated by coughing, bending or sudden movements
subarachnoid hemorrhage	◊ **sudden onset** ("worst ever")

IMPLEMENTATION
- Obtain history, trigger factors, medications
- Reduce environmental stimuli
- Watch for signs of increased intracranial pressure
- Teach client ways to reduce stress

MIGRAINE:
- Avoid cheese and red wine
- Teach client to take ergotamine as early as possible during acute attack

13.8.) <u>INCREASED INTRACRANIAL PRESSURE</u>

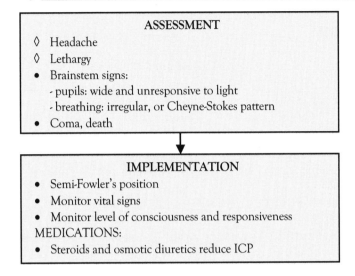

ASSESSMENT
- ◊ Headache
- ◊ Lethargy
- Brainstem signs:
  - pupils: wide and unresponsive to light
  - breathing: irregular, or Cheyne-Stokes pattern
- Coma, death

IMPLEMENTATION
- Semi-Fowler's position
- Monitor vital signs
- Monitor level of consciousness and responsiveness
MEDICATIONS:
- Steroids and osmotic diuretics reduce ICP

13.9.) <u>MENINGITIS</u>

ASSESSMENT
- ◊ Headache, backache
- ◊ Lethargy
- Fever
- Nuchal rigidity
- **Kernig's sign:** Extend client's legs. Positive if pain or spasm occurs
- **Brudzinski's sign:** Flex neck. Positive if client flexes hip and knees
- Diagnosis: Lumbar puncture, CSF

ANALYSIS
- Risk of cerebral edema and permanent damage

IMPLEMENTATION
- Monitor vital signs and level of consciousness frequently
- Monitor central venous pressure
- Keep room dark if client is photophobic
- Close contacts may need Rifampin prophylaxis

13.10.) STROKE

TIA	• <u>transient</u> focal neurologic deficits • lasts minutes to hours • leaves no residual effect
ischemic	• **embolic or thrombotic occlusion** <u>RISK FACTORS</u>: - arteriosclerosis - atrial fibrillation - disease of heart valves
hemorrhagic	• **rupture of cerebral blood vessel** <u>RISK FACTORS</u>: - intracranial aneurysms - arteriovenous malformations - hypertension

TIA = *transient ischemic attack, due to microthrombi*

ASSESSMENT

◊ Sudden numbness or muscle weakness
◊ Dizziness
◊ Difficulty speaking
- **Parietal cortex:** Hemiparesis
  - occurs on opposite side of body
- **Temporal cortex:** Aphasia
  - difficulty speaking or understanding language or both
- **Occipital cortex:** Visual defects
- **Cerebellum:** Vertigo, ataxia

IMPLEMENTATION

- Maintain bed rest
- Maintain open airways
- Position client on side if unconscious (to prevent aspiration)
- Monitor vital signs and neurological status
- Monitor for signs of increased intracranial pressure
- Meticulous skin care, turn client frequently

PHYSICAL ACTIVITY:

- Encourage activities: begin rehabilitation immediately
- Physical therapy & Speech therapy

PROPER POSITION:

- Use trochanter roll to prevent external rotation of hip
- Use bed board to keep foot dorsiflexed
- Put small pillow in axilla to prevent shoulder adduction
- Slightly elevate hand to prevent edema

Client with aphasia:
1. Speak at normal rate and volume (client's hearing is intact).
2. Ask questions that require simple answers.
3. Allow time for response, do not press for answers.
4. Observe nonverbal clues.

13.11.) PARAPLEGIA / QUADRIPLEGIA

> **Paraplegia:** spinal cord trauma at thoracic or lumbar level
> **Quadriplegia:** spinal cord trauma at cervical level

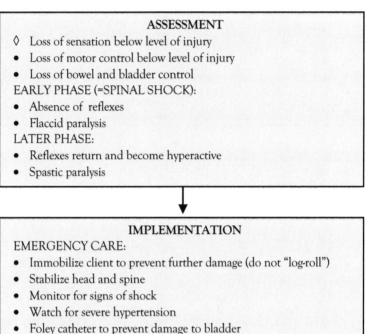

ASSESSMENT
◊ Loss of sensation below level of injury
- Loss of motor control below level of injury
- Loss of bowel and bladder control
EARLY PHASE (=SPINAL SHOCK):
- Absence of reflexes
- Flaccid paralysis
LATER PHASE:
- Reflexes return and become hyperactive
- Spastic paralysis

IMPLEMENTATION
EMERGENCY CARE:
- Immobilize client to prevent further damage (do not "log-roll")
- Stabilize head and spine
- Monitor for signs of shock
- Watch for severe hypertension
- Foley catheter to prevent damage to bladder
LATER PHASE:
- Use intermittent catheterization
- Monitor fluid intake / output
- Monitor for signs of urinary tract infection
- Meticulous skin care, turn client frequently

CLIENT EDUCATION
- Automatic bladder: Teach client how to initiate urination
- Sex education and counseling

13.12.) PERIPHERAL NEUROPATHIES

CAUSES:

toxins	- lead - arsenic - mercury - many drugs
nutritional	- vit. B1 deficiency - vit. B6 deficiency - vit. B12 deficiency
other acquired	- Guillain-Barré syndrome *(follows viral infection)* - amyotrophic lateral sclerosis - diabetes mellitus

*Peripheral neuropathy **in alcoholics** is usually due to thiamin (vitamin B1) or cobalamin (vitamin B12) deficiency.*

B12 deficiency also causes megaloblastic anemia in these clients.

13.13.) PARKINSON'S DISEASE

Damage to dopaminergic neurons in the *substantia nigra* of the brainstem

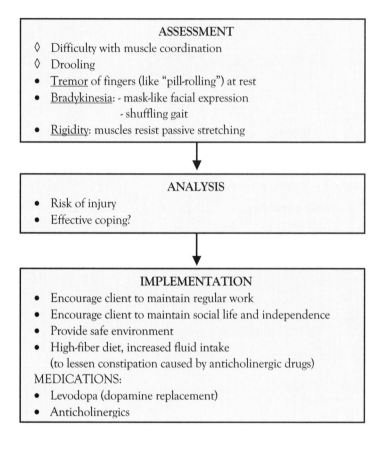

ASSESSMENT
◊ Difficulty with muscle coordination
◊ Drooling
● <u>Tremor</u> of fingers (like "pill-rolling") at rest
● <u>Bradykinesia</u>: - mask-like facial expression
               - shuffling gait
● <u>Rigidity</u>: muscles resist passive stretching

ANALYSIS
● Risk of injury
● Effective coping?

IMPLEMENTATION
● Encourage client to maintain regular work
● Encourage client to maintain social life and independence
● Provide safe environment
● High-fiber diet, increased fluid intake
  (to lessen constipation caused by anticholinergic drugs)
MEDICATIONS:
● Levodopa (dopamine replacement)
● Anticholinergics

"On-off" phenomenon: Abrupt transient changes in severity of symptoms occurring unpredictably during the day. (Late complication after years of treatment.)

13.14.) MULTIPLE SCLEROSIS

Progressive patchy demyelination of white matter of CNS

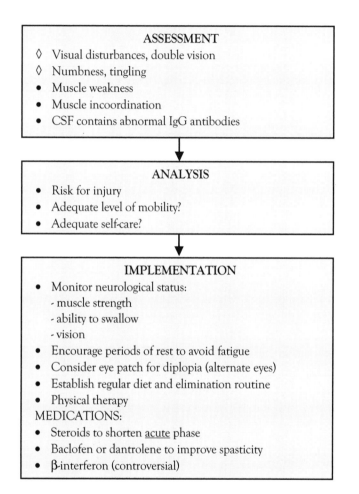

ASSESSMENT
- ◊ Visual disturbances, double vision
- ◊ Numbness, tingling
- Muscle weakness
- Muscle incoordination
- CSF contains abnormal IgG antibodies

ANALYSIS
- Risk for injury
- Adequate level of mobility?
- Adequate self-care?

IMPLEMENTATION
- Monitor neurological status:
  - muscle strength
  - ability to swallow
  - vision
- Encourage periods of rest to avoid fatigue
- Consider eye patch for diplopia (alternate eyes)
- Establish regular diet and elimination routine
- Physical therapy

MEDICATIONS:
- Steroids to shorten <u>acute</u> phase
- Baclofen or dantrolene to improve spasticity
- β-interferon (controversial)

13.15.) <u>AMYOTROPHIC LATERAL SCLEROSIS</u>
Progressive degeneration of motor neurons

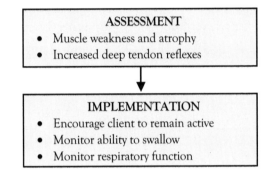

ASSESSMENT
- Muscle weakness and atrophy
- Increased deep tendon reflexes

IMPLEMENTATION
- Encourage client to remain active
- Monitor ability to swallow
- Monitor respiratory function

13.16.) <u>BELL'S PALSY</u>
Paralysis of one side of face, usually due to inflammation of 7th cranial nerve

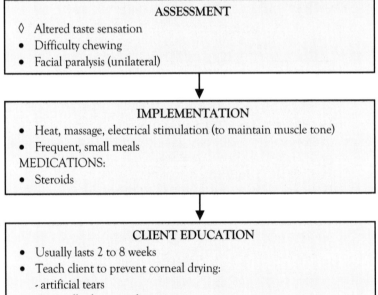

ASSESSMENT
- ◊ Altered taste sensation
- Difficulty chewing
- Facial paralysis (unilateral)

IMPLEMENTATION
- Heat, massage, electrical stimulation (to maintain muscle tone)
- Frequent, small meals
MEDICATIONS:
- Steroids

CLIENT EDUCATION
- Usually lasts 2 to 8 weeks
- Teach client to prevent corneal drying:
  - artificial tears
  - manually close eye if necessary

13.17.) EPILEPSY

grand mal	◊ loss of consciousness • tonic, then clonic • incontinence
petit mal	◊ absence seizure ("blank spell") • no loss of muscle tone
narcolepsy	• REM onset sleep • loss of muscle tone
psychomotor	• non-goal directed activity (lip smacking, walking...)
Jacksonian	• spreading muscle group activity (e.g. fingers → forearm → shoulder)

IMPLEMENTATION
DURING SEIZURE:
- Maintain patent airways
- Protect client from injury
- Do not restrain

AFTER SEIZURE:
- Bed rest with padded side rails
- Keep diazepam ("Valium") and oxygen at bedside

CLIENT EDUCATION
- Teach importance to comply with medications
- Never abruptly discontinue anticonvulsants
- Abstain from alcohol

DISEASES
OF THE
EYES & EARS

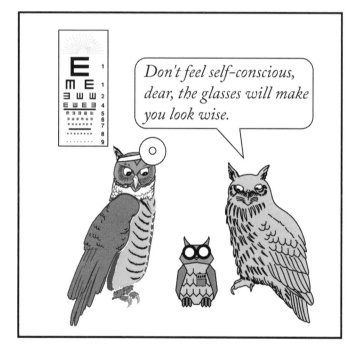

14.1.) REFRACTION

myopic eye   corrected with negative lens

hypermetropic eye   corrected with positive lens

myopia (nearsightedness)	- lens has normal elasticity - eye ball too long (or focal point too short)
hypermetropia [1] (farsightedness)	- lens has normal elasticity - eye ball too short (or focal point too far) - don't confuse with presbyopia
presbyopia [1] (age)	- lens has lost elasticity - cannot shorten focal length - *corrected with positive lens*

[1] both have difficulty reading

 A client with 20/30 vision can read letter of size 30 from a distance of 20 feet (i.e. cannot read smaller sizes 20 or 10).

14.2.) <u>CATARACT</u>
Clouding of lens → decreased light transmission

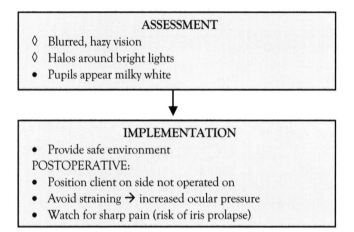

ASSESSMENT
◊ Blurred, hazy vision
◊ Halos around bright lights
• Pupils appear milky white

IMPLEMENTATION
• Provide safe environment
POSTOPERATIVE:
• Position client on side not operated on
• Avoid straining → increased ocular pressure
• Watch for sharp pain (risk of iris prolapse)

14.3.) <u>BLINDNESS</u>

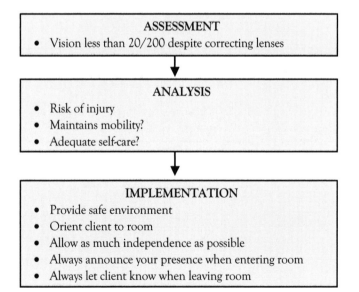

ASSESSMENT
• Vision less than 20/200 despite correcting lenses

ANALYSIS
• Risk of injury
• Maintains mobility?
• Adequate self-care?

IMPLEMENTATION
• Provide safe environment
• Orient client to room
• Allow as much independence as possible
• Always announce your presence when entering room
• Always let client know when leaving room

14.4.) CONJUNCTIVITIS

	ALLERGIC	BACTERIAL	VIRAL
itching	severe	little	little
injection	mild	severe	moderate
discharge	mild	severe	moderate
lymph nodes	negative	negative	enlarged
often associated with	hay fever	-	sore throat
MEDICATIONS:	steroids antihistamines	topical antibiotics	-

14.5.) CHALAZION & STYE

➤ **Chalazion** = internal hordeolum (inflammation of Meibomian gland)
➤ **Stye** = external hordeolum (inflammation of glands of Zeiss or Moll)

ASSESSMENT
◊ Pain
◊ Foreign body sensation
• Sty: pain and redness of lid margin → small tender induration, pus
• Chalazion: lid edema, subconjunctival mass

↓

IMPLEMENTATION
• Warm compresses
MEDICATIONS:
• Topical antibiotics

216

14.6.) <u>GLAUCOMA</u>

Abnormal increase in intraocular pressure → medical emergency!

open angle (chronic)	◊ asymptomatic until late stage • gradual loss of peripheral vision ("tunnel vision")
closed angle (acute)	◊ severe eye pain ◊ blurred vision ◊ headache • reddened eye • dilated, non-reactive pupils - due to blockage of aqueous drainage - may be precipitated by pupil dilation (atropine)

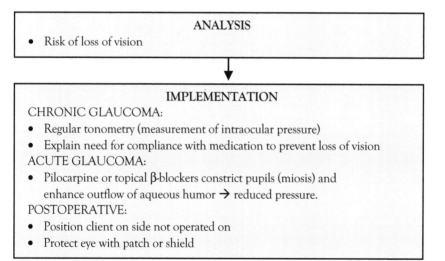

ANALYSIS

• Risk of loss of vision

↓

IMPLEMENTATION

CHRONIC GLAUCOMA:
• Regular tonometry (measurement of intraocular pressure)
• Explain need for compliance with medication to prevent loss of vision
ACUTE GLAUCOMA:
• Pilocarpine or topical β-blockers constrict pupils (miosis) and enhance outflow of aqueous humor → reduced pressure.
POSTOPERATIVE:
• Position client on side not operated on
• Protect eye with patch or shield

14.7.) <u>RETINA DETACHMENT</u>

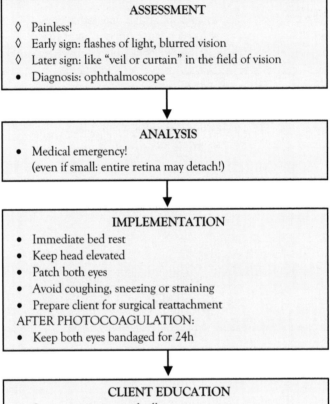

ASSESSMENT
◊ Painless!
◊ Early sign: flashes of light, blurred vision
◊ Later sign: like "veil or curtain" in the field of vision
• Diagnosis: ophthalmoscope

ANALYSIS
• Medical emergency!
  (even if small: entire retina may detach!)

IMPLEMENTATION
• Immediate bed rest
• Keep head elevated
• Patch both eyes
• Avoid coughing, sneezing or straining
• Prepare client for surgical reattachment
AFTER PHOTOCOAGULATION:
• Keep both eyes bandaged for 24h

CLIENT EDUCATION
• Resume activities gradually
• Immediately seek help if symptoms reoccur

14.8.) ASSESSMENT: EARS

hearing loss	**CONDUCTIVE HEARING LOSS (damage to outer ear or middle ear):** - cerumen - tympanic membrane perforation - otitis media - otosclerosis **SENSORINEURAL HEARING LOSS (damage to inner ear):** - presbyacusis - ototoxic drugs: aminoglycosides - Ménière's disease - acoustic neurinoma
tinnitus ("ear ringing")	**CAUSED BY DRUGS:** - salicylates, quinine, aminoglycosides **CAUSED BY DISEASES:** - hypertension - labyrinthitis - Ménière's disease - acoustic neurinoma

14.9.) OTOSCLEROSIS

Degeneration of bones in the middle ear

ASSESSMENT

- Progressive hearing loss (often in young adults)
- Weber test: sound lateralizes to sick ear
  (hold tuning fork on top of skull and ask client which side
  she hears the sound)

↓

IMPLEMENTATION

- Monitor degree of hearing loss
- Prepare client for surgery (*stapes* is replaced by prosthesis)

POSTOPERATIVE:

- Refrain from blowing nose for 1 week
- Avoid pressure changes (flying or diving)

14.10.) PRESBYACUSIS

Hearing loss occurring as part of normal aging

ASSESSMENT

- Highest tones are lost first!
- Client's own speech is louder than average
- Client may become angry or depressed

↓

IMPLEMENTATION

- Reduce distracting background noises
- Face client when speaking
- Encourage client to use hearing aid

14.11.) <u>MÉNIÈRE'S DISEASE</u>
Inner ear disease of unknown cause

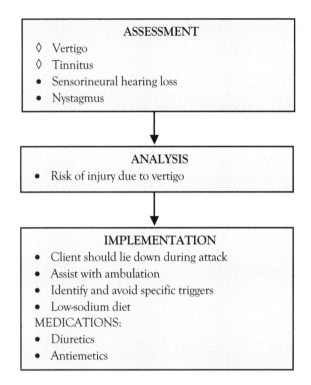

ASSESSMENT
◊ Vertigo
◊ Tinnitus
• Sensorineural hearing loss
• Nystagmus

ANALYSIS
• Risk of injury due to vertigo

IMPLEMENTATION
• Client should lie down during attack
• Assist with ambulation
• Identify and avoid specific triggers
• Low-sodium diet
MEDICATIONS:
• Diuretics
• Antiemetics

Surgical destruction of labyrinth or vestibular nerve abolishes vertigo but unfortunately will also cause deafness.

➢ **Vertigo** = feeling that the room is spinning

DISEASES
OF THE SKIN

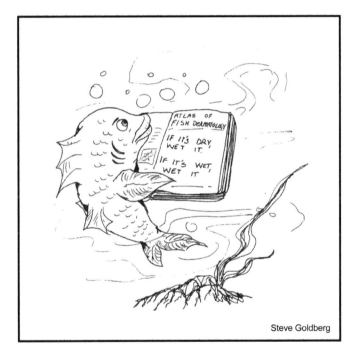

Steve Goldberg

15.1.) SKIN LESIONS

A) PRIMARY LESIONS:

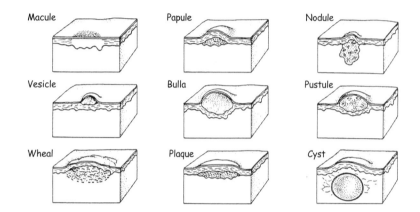

B) SECONDARY LESIONS:

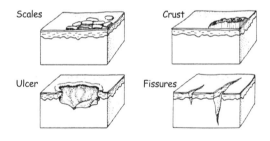

15.2.) DERMATITIS

acute contact dermatitis
"a rash that itches"

CLIENT EDUCATION
- **avoid irritants**
  - soap, detergents
- **avoid allergens**
  - poison ivy, metals, drugs

---

atopic dermatitis
"an itch that rashes"

ASSESSMENT
◊ a/w asthma, hay fever
◊ worsened by stress, premenstrual
- papules, vesicles, crusts
LOCATIONS:
- cheeks, scalp, neck
- flexor surfaces of arms or legs

CLIENT EDUCATION
- avoid scratching (infants may need to be restrained)
- avoid wool clothing and blankets
- keep skin hydrated

---

seborrheic dermatitis

ASSESSMENT
- scaly, oily patches
- slight erythema at base
LOCATIONS:
- scalp
- eye brows
- retroauricular
- presternal

CLIENT EDUCATION
- use daily zinc, selenium, sulfur or tar shampoos
- use topical hydrocortisone if necessary
- avoid fluorinated corticosteroids (risk of skin atrophy)

15.3.) ACNE

ASSESSMENT
- Closed comedones ("whiteheads")
- Open comedones ("blackheads")
- Papules / pustules

IMPLEMENTATION
MEDICATIONS:
- Benzoyl peroxide
- Retinoic acid cream, antibiotics

CLIENT EDUCATION
- Wash face gently with mild soap, 1-2 times daily
- Never squeeze pimples
- Retinoic acid (Accutane) may cause birth defects!
  (→ use contraceptives when on Accutane)

15.4.) SEBORRHEIC ECZEMA

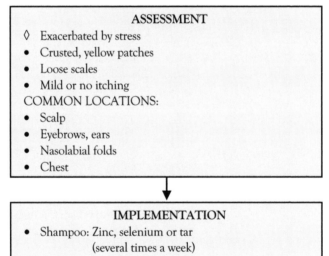

ASSESSMENT
- ◊ Exacerbated by stress
- Crusted, yellow patches
- Loose scales
- Mild or no itching
COMMON LOCATIONS:
- Scalp
- Eyebrows, ears
- Nasolabial folds
- Chest

IMPLEMENTATION
- Shampoo: Zinc, selenium or tar
  (several times a week)
- Corticosteroid lotions or creams

15.5.) **PSORIASIS**

Chronic inflammatory skin disease with extremely rapid epidermal turnover

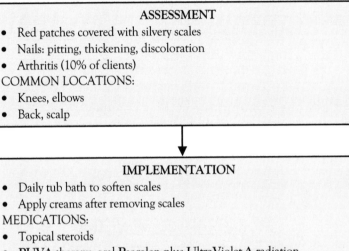

ASSESSMENT
- Red patches covered with silvery scales
- Nails: pitting, thickening, discoloration
- Arthritis (10% of clients)

COMMON LOCATIONS:
- Knees, elbows
- Back, scalp

IMPLEMENTATION
- Daily tub bath to soften scales
- Apply creams after removing scales

MEDICATIONS:
- Topical steroids
- **PUVA** therapy: oral **P**soralen plus **U**ltra**V**iolet-**A** radiation photosensitization lasts full day: wear sunscreen outdoors!

Köbner phenomenon: *Lesions tend to appear at sites of minor trauma.*

15.6.) <u>STASIS DERMATITIS</u>

Caused by venous stasis and chronic thrombophlebitis

ASSESSMENT
- ◊ Itching skin
- Typically located just above medial malleolus
- Brown skin discoloration (deposition of hemosiderin)
- Ulceration

IMPLEMENTATION
- Leg elevation to decrease edema
- Compression bandage
- Surgical removal of varicose veins

15.7.) <u>VARICOSE VEINS</u>

ASSESSMENT
- ◊ Cramping, pain in legs
- Foot and ankle edema
- Pigmentation of ankles and calves

ANALYSIS
- Decreased comfort due to swelling and pain

IMPLEMENTATION
- Avoid prolonged standing
- Avoid sitting cross-legged
- Rest with legs elevated
- Support stockings

VARICOSECTOMY:
- Watch for bleeding
- Watch for thrombophlebitis → calf pain
- Assess potential damage to saphenous nerve
  (→ sensory loss at medial side of leg)

15.8.) SKIN TUMORS

	ASSESSMENT
seborrheic keratosis "senile warts"	◊ very common in the elderly • benign epidermal tumors • multiple occurrence • usually pigmented, scaly
actinic keratosis	• scaly red patches on sun exposed areas • may develop into squamous cell carcinoma (risk about 1%)
squamous cell carcinoma	• ulcerated erosion or nodule
basal cell carcinoma	• translucent, pearly white appearance • raised borders • may be ulcerated • bleeds easily
malignant melanoma	**The ABC of melanoma:** - **A**symmetrical - **B**orders irregular, notched - **C**olor: various shades of brown - **D**iameter increasing

Avoid sunburns, especially at young age !

INJURY

&

POISONING

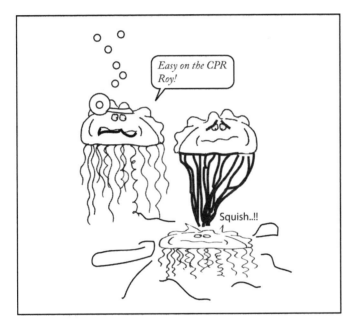

16.1.) <u>ABC OF TRAUMA</u>

1. AIRWAYS

- Jaw-thrust maneuver:
  - move mandible forward while tilting head backward
  - don't tilt head in case of suspected cervical spine injury
- Remove mucus, broken teeth, dentures from mouth

2. BREATHING

- Note breathing pattern: regularity, frequency
- Assess for pneumothorax: auscultate or percuss both lungs
- Assess for tension pneumothorax: trachea deviates to healthy side
- Ventilation, oxygen

3. CIRCULATION

- Cardiac arrest: start chest compression and ventilation
- Apply pressure over bleeding sites
- Femur fractures and pelvic trauma can cause massive internal bleeding
- Monitor for signs of shock → Trendelenburg position

Assume cervical spine injury in <u>every</u> unconscious trauma victim until ruled out.

16.2.) POISONING

IMPLEMENTATION
- Gastric lavage if within 2h of ingestion
- **Induced vomiting is NOT recommended anymore**
- Activated charcoal to minimize gastrointestinal absorption
- Monitor vital signs and level of consciousness
- Specific antidotes (see below):

INTOXICATION	ANTIDOTE
methanol, ethylene glycol	ethanol
acetaminophen	N-acetylcysteine
benzodiazepines	flumazenil
opiates	naloxone
carbon monoxide	100% oxygen
cyanide	amyl nitrate
iron	deferoxamine
lead	EDTA
Warfarin	vitamin K
heparin	protamine

16.3.) HEAD TRAUMA

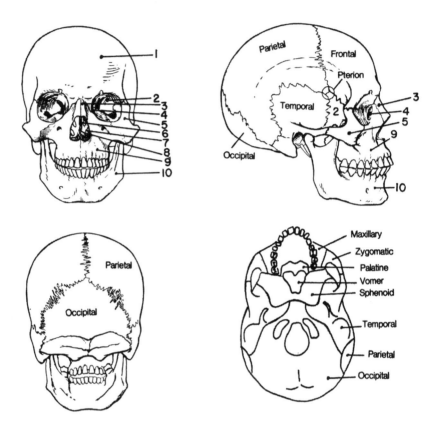

From Goldberg: *Clinical Anatomy Made Ridiculously Simple*, MedMaster, 2007

1	frontal bone	6	ethmoid bone
2	sphenoid bone	7	inferior nasal conch
3	nasal bone	8	vomer
4	lacrimal bone	9	maxilla
5	zygomatic bone	10	mandible

	SIGNS & SYMPTOMS
concussion	◊ brief loss of consciousness ◊ transient amnesia (anterograde and retrograde) • no identifiable neuropathological changes • **CT scan normal**
contusion	• cerebral edema • diffuse intracerebral hemorrhage • if localized: **focal neurological signs** • if generalized: focal signs plus mental impairment
epidural hematoma	◊ momentary unconsciousness followed by: ◊ **lucid interval** for a few hours, followed by: ◊ headache, vomiting, rapidly decreasing level of consciousness
subdural hematoma	◊ **delayed** for days or weeks after injury (occasionally may be acute) - more common in elderly and alcoholics
basilar skull fractures	• hemotympanum • mastoid ecchymosis • periorbital ecchymosis • facial palsy • CSF in nasal secretion

ASSESSMENT

◊ Irritability, confusion
◊ Behavioral changes
   (client may be combative or indifferent)
◊ Decreased level of consciousness
• Nausea, vomiting

FOCAL SIGNS:

• Paralysis on side opposite to brain injury
• Sensory loss on side opposite to brain injury

BRAIN-STEM INJURY:

• Large pupils, loss of light reflex
• Loss of gag reflex

ANALYSIS

• Adequate cerebral perfusion?
• Adequate cardiac output?
• Complications of immobility?

IMPLEMENTATION

• Concussion: Careful observation!
   (if neurological signs → needs to be admitted)

• Maintain airway patency
• Stabilize cervical injury
• Monitor for signs of increased intracranial pressure
• Monitor for CSF leakage from nose

• Monitor vital signs
• Monitor breathing pattern
• Use Glasgow coma scale

16.4.) CHEST TRAUMA

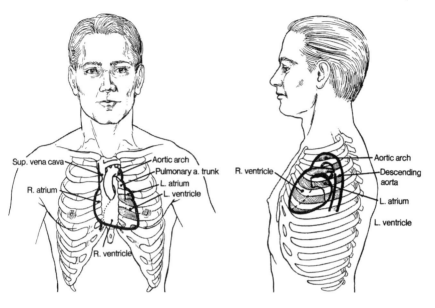

From Goldberg: *Clinical Anatomy Made Ridiculously Simple*, MedMaster, 2007

A) CARDIOVASCULAR:

cardiac tamponade (penetrating chest trauma)	• hypotension • jugular vein distention (unless patient is severely hypovolemic)
aortic dissection (often fatal)	• progressive hypotension and shock • mediastinal widening
hemothorax (penetrating or blunt trauma)	• shock, hypotension • often combined with pneumothorax

237

B) PULMONARY:

pneumothorax (spontaneous or after trauma)	◊ sudden chest pain • hyperresonance
tension pneumothorax (rapidly fatal unless treated)	◊ sudden chest pain, • hyperresonance • ventilatory and circulatory compromise • mediastinal shift to healthy side
open pneumothorax (due to penetrating injury)	- small wounds may create tension pneumothorax (valve-like mechanism)
pulmonary contusion (a/w rib fractures)	• hypoxemia • pulmonary infiltrates on chest X-ray
flail chest (multiple rib fractures)	• unstable segment moves inward during inspiration ("paradoxical movement") • respiratory distress

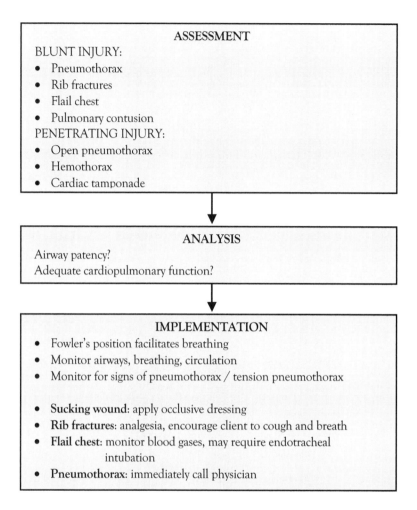

ASSESSMENT

BLUNT INJURY:
- Pneumothorax
- Rib fractures
- Flail chest
- Pulmonary contusion

PENETRATING INJURY:
- Open pneumothorax
- Hemothorax
- Cardiac tamponade

ANALYSIS

Airway patency?
Adequate cardiopulmonary function?

IMPLEMENTATION
- Fowler's position facilitates breathing
- Monitor airways, breathing, circulation
- Monitor for signs of pneumothorax / tension pneumothorax

- **Sucking wound:** apply occlusive dressing
- **Rib fractures:** analgesia, encourage client to cough and breath
- **Flail chest:** monitor blood gases, may require endotracheal intubation
- **Pneumothorax:** immediately call physician

Tension pneumothorax → *prepare to convert to open pneumothorax.*

239

16.5.) ABDOMINAL TRAUMA

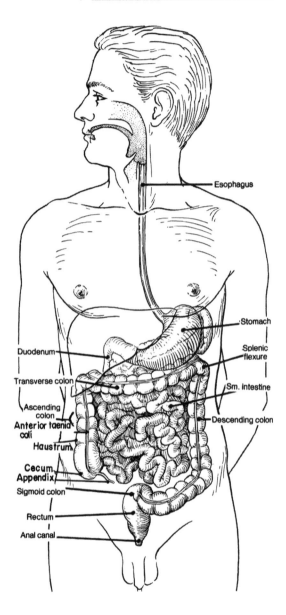

From Goldberg: *Clinical Anatomy Made Ridiculously Simple*, MedMaster, 2007

240

hemorrhage	**liver, spleen, major vessel injury** - suspect in all clients with abdominal trauma and shock!
peritonitis	**intestinal and pancreatic injury** • fever, tachycardia, diffuse pain, ileus
spleen rupture	**most common injury of <u>blunt</u> abdominal trauma** ◊ left upper quadrant pain ◊ may radiate to shoulder • intra-abdominal hemorrhage (shock, hypotension, peritoneal signs)
liver injury	**most common injury of <u>penetrating</u> abdominal trauma** ◊ right upper quadrant pain • intra-abdominal hemorrhage (shock, hypotension, peritoneal signs)
intestinal injury	**usually due to penetrating trauma** - small intestinal injury is more common - large intestinal injury is more severe • signs of peritonitis (rebound tenderness, muscle rigidity)

IMPLEMENTATION
- Do not attempt to replace protruding organs: cover with sterile saline dressing instead
- IV fluids (oral fluids may cause vomiting)
- Assist with peritoneal lavage
- Monitor vital signs, bowel sounds and urinary output

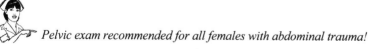

Pelvic exam recommended for all females with abdominal trauma!

16.6.) <u>GENITOURINARY TRAUMA</u>

<u>FEMALE</u>:

<u>MALE</u>:

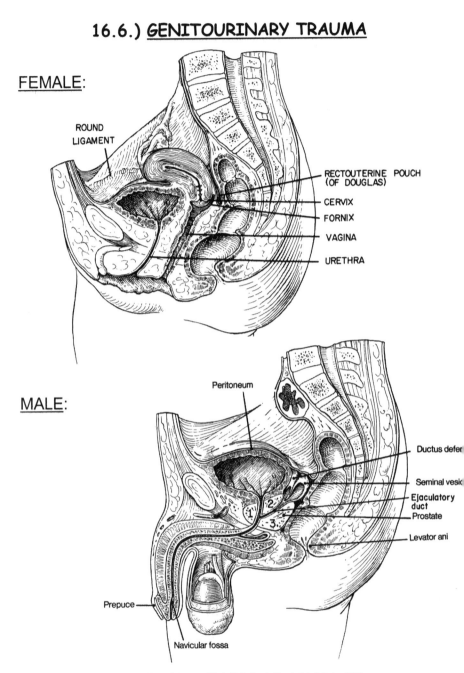

From Goldberg: *Clinical Anatomy Made Ridiculously Simple*, MedMaster, 2007

bladder rupture	- common with pelvic fractures • gross hematuria (obtain urine sample via catheter) • intraperitoneal rupture → acute abdomen
urethra rupture	• may result in impotence and incontinence • bloody urethral discharge
kidney injury	- common in motor vehicle accidents • lower rib fractures • flank pain

 Monitor patients with pelvic trauma for hemorrhagic shock.
Internal bleeding can be massive!

16.7.) FRACTURES

A) LOCATIONS:

	KEY FEATURES
hip	- osteoporosis is a major risk factor!
ribs	- **pain that worsens with deep breathing** - flail chest: inward movement of rib cage during inspiration
Colle's	- fracture and displacement of distal radius - **results from fall on outstretched hand**
elbow	- more common in children - watch for injury of median nerve and radial artery - **avoid Volkmann's contracture** (ischemic damage)
pelvis	- most commonly due to motor vehicle accident - **risk of major internal blood loss!**
tibia	- **risk of compartment syndrome**
Pott's	- fracture of distal fibula and torn off internal malleolus - **results from foot eversion and abduction**

B) TYPES:

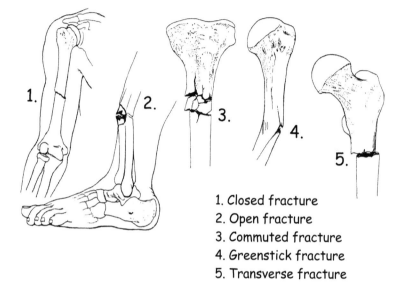

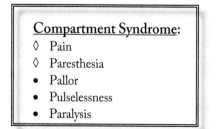

1. Closed fracture
2. Open fracture
3. Commuted fracture
4. Greenstick fracture
5. Transverse fracture

Volkmann's Contracture:

Tight cast → compartment syndrome → irreversible nerve / muscle damage

---

Compartment Syndrome:
◊ Pain
◊ Paresthesia
• Pallor
• Pulselessness
• Paralysis

C) MANAGEMENT:

clavicle	- posterior T-splint
humerus	- hanging cast - exercise to prevent stiffening of shoulder - watch for signs of Volkmann's ischemic contracture
radius, ulna	- closed (or open) reduction, intraosseous pins
cervical vertebrae	- if suspected: immobilize immediately
pelvis	- requires 6~8 weeks bed rest
femur neck	- common site of non-union - avoid abduction plaster cast (better: internal fixation)
tibia (±fibula)	- plaster splint
Pott's	- closed reduction, plaster cast

16.8.) SPRAINS

IMPLEMENTATION
- RICE = Rest, Ice, Compression, Elevation
- Knee joint: early mobilization is important

MEDICATIONS:
- NSAIDs

16.9.) <u>NERVE INJURIES</u>

DAMAGE TO :	RESULTS IN IMPAIRED FUNCTION OF:
axillary nerve	shoulder abduction
musculocutaneous nerve	elbow flexion
* radial nerve	finger and wrist extension [1] *(= "wrist drop")*
* median nerve	flexion of first 3 fingers [2] *(= "carpal tunnel syndrome")*
ulnar nerve	finger and thumb adduction [3] *(= "claw hand")*
femoral nerve	knee extension
superior gluteal nerve	hip abduction
inferior gluteal nerve	hip extension
tibial nerve	foot plantar flexion
* peroneal nerve	foot dorsiflexion and eversion [4] *(= "foot drop")*

* = easily damaged in clients with casts

[1] Have client extend fingers - check sensation of dorsal web between thumb and 2nd finger.

[2] Have client touch palm with index finger - check palmar sensation of first 3 fingers.

[3] Have client touch 5th finger with thumb - check sensation of 5th and lateral 4th fingers.

[4] Have client point toe upward (towards nose) - check sensation on dorsum of foot.

MAIN NERVES OF ARM:

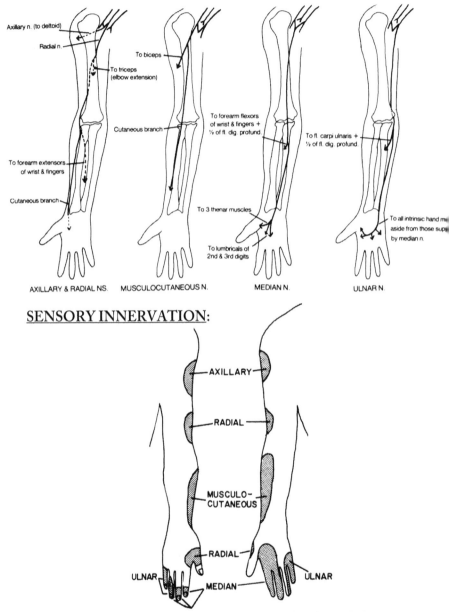

Axillary n. (to deltoid)

Radial n.

To biceps

To triceps
(elbow extension)

Cutaneous branch

To forearm flexors
of wrist & fingers +
½ of fl. dig. profund.

To fl. carpi ulnaris +
½ of fl. dig. profund.

To forearm extensors
of wrist & fingers

Cutaneous branch

To 3 thenar muscles

To all intrinsic hand m
aside from those sup
by median n.

To lumbricals of
2nd & 3rd digits

AXILLARY & RADIAL NS.   MUSCULOCUTANEOUS N.   MEDIAN N.   ULNAR N.

SENSORY INNERVATION:

AXILLARY

RADIAL

MUSCULO-
CUTANEOUS

RADIAL

ULNAR   ULNAR

MEDIAN

From Goldberg: *Clinical Anatomy Made Ridiculously Simple*, MedMaster, 2007

MAIN NERVES OF LEG:

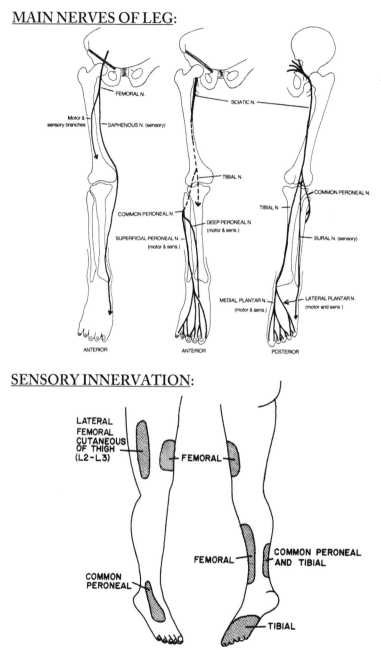

SENSORY INNERVATION:

From Goldberg: *Clinical Anatomy Made Ridiculously Simple*, MedMaster, 2007

16.10.) <u>CASTS</u>

- ➢ immobilize fractured bones
- ➢ stabilize weak joints
- ➢ permit early mobilization

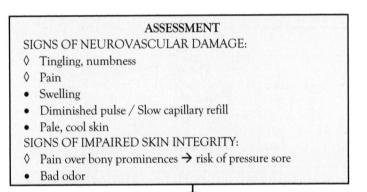

ASSESSMENT
SIGNS OF NEUROVASCULAR DAMAGE:
- ◊ Tingling, numbness
- ◊ Pain
- • Swelling
- • Diminished pulse / Slow capillary refill
- • Pale, cool skin
SIGNS OF IMPAIRED SKIN INTEGRITY:
- ◊ Pain over bony prominences → risk of pressure sore
- • Bad odor

ANALYSIS
- • Adequate tissue perfusion?
- • Impaired physical mobility?

IMPLEMENTATION
FRESH CAST:
- • Monitor neurovascular status hourly for first 24h.
- • Handle moist cast with <u>palms of hands</u> (not fingers)
- • Reduce swelling: ice packs, elevation
CONTINUED CARE:
- • Range of motion exercises
- • Isometric exercises for the muscles inside cast
- • Signs of neurovascular damage: split cast in half and
                              cut underlying padding

CLIENT EDUCATION
- • Encourage client to elevate cast frequently
- • Avoid weight bearing on cast during first 24 hours
- • Avoid wetting cast

16.11.) <u>TRACTION</u>

ASSESSMENT

COMPLICATIONS:
- Skin breakdown under traction
- Infection along pin tracts
- Complications of immobility

IMPLEMENTATION
- Assess equipment
  - weights should hang freely
  - ropes should be in line with extremities
- Exercise uninvolved muscles and joints
- Monitor for signs of infection: redness and drainage at pin site
- Assess for signs of thrombophlebitis
- Provide regular back care, back rubs

Buck's traction:
➤ Provides immobility and support (temporary measure only)
➤ Use foam traction boot or traction tape
➤ Requires, clean, dry, healthy skin

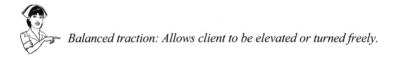

Balanced traction: Allows client to be elevated or turned freely.

External fixation:
➤ For open fractures and infected nonunions
➤ Facilitates wound care, debridement, dressing changes
➤ Watch for signs of infection around pins

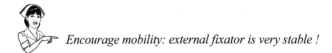

Encourage mobility: external fixator is very stable !

251

16.12.) <u>BURNS</u>

EXTENT:

> *Rule of 9:* The body is divided into 11 areas, each representing 9% of surface.

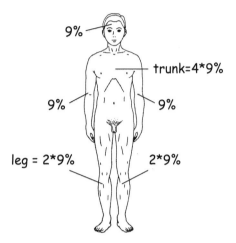

9%

trunk=4*9%

9%   9%

leg = 2*9%   2*9%

DEGREE:

First degree	- pink to red - mild edema - *no scarring*
Second degree	- pink to red, blanches on pressure - blister formation - hair does not pull out easily - *scarring possible*
Third degree	- reddened areas don't blanch to pressure - formation of devitalized, leathery tissue - hair pulls out easily - *scarring expected*

ASSESSMENT

- Determine degree
- Determine extent

SIGNS OF CO TOXICITY:
◊ Headache, irritability, confusion
◊ Muscular fatigue
- Nausea, vomiting
- Convulsions, coma, death

EMERGENCY CARE

- First aid **ABC**
- Prevent shock
- IV fluids to maintain urine output > 0.5 mL/kg/h
  Crystalloids: Salt solutions (for example Ringer's lactate)
  Colloids: Contains large organic molecules (for example albumin)
- Treat respiratory distress

ACUTE CARE

- NPO for first 24h, assess bowel sounds (paralytic ileus is common)
- Monitor ECG (risk of arrhythmia due to electrolyte imbalance)
- Watch for signs of infection and sepsis
- High-protein, high-calorie diet

WOUND CARE:
- Cleanse wounds and change dressing twice daily
- Non-viable tissue ("eschar") should be removed
- Topical antimicrobial creams or ointments
- Maintain asepsis!

REHABILITATION

- Prevent contractures
- Provide counseling

Half of all fire deaths are due to inhalation of smoke and CO.

16.13.) DROWNING

ASSESSMENT
COMPLICATIONS:
- ARDS (acute respiratory distress syndrome)
- Cerebral edema
- Cardiac arrhythmias due to electrolyte imbalance

IMPLEMENTATION
- "The client isn't dead until she is warm and dead" because immersion in cold water slows brain metabolism
- Resuscitate immediately
- Do not waste time attempting to drain water from victims lungs or stomach

- Monitor ECG
- Monitor for pulmonary complications

CLIENT EDUCATION
- Drowning is a common cause of accidents in children
- Provide close supervision around swimming pools!

16.14.) <u>ALTITUDE SICKNESS</u>

Low oxygen → hyperventilation → respiratory alkalosis

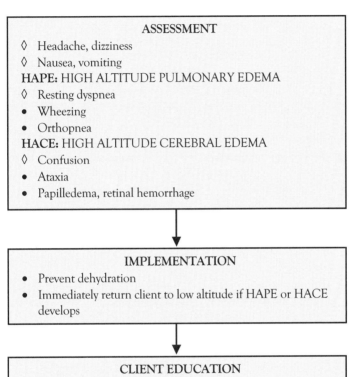

ASSESSMENT
◊ Headache, dizziness
◊ Nausea, vomiting
HAPE: HIGH ALTITUDE PULMONARY EDEMA
◊ Resting dyspnea
• Wheezing
• Orthopnea
HACE: HIGH ALTITUDE CEREBRAL EDEMA
◊ Confusion
• Ataxia
• Papilledema, retinal hemorrhage

IMPLEMENTATION
• Prevent dehydration
• Immediately return client to low altitude if HAPE or HACE develops

CLIENT EDUCATION
• Slow ascent allows gradual acclimatization
• Acetazolamide is an effective prophylactic

16.15.) BITES & STINGS

Animal Bites:

> Risk of infection: Monkey > Cat > Dog bites

IMPLEMENTATION
- Cleanse, débride and irrigate wound
- Hospitalize if infection involves hand
- Consider rabies prophylaxis

Spider Bites:

ASSESSMENT

BLACK WIDOW:
- Abdominal pain
- Vomiting
- Shock

BROWN RECLUSIVE SPIDER:
- Fever, rash
- Jaundice

Insect Stings:

IMPLEMENTATION
- Ice packs to relieve pain
- Oral steroids if large local reaction

ANAPHYLAXIS:
- Have epinephrine and antihistamines on hand

CLIENT EDUCATION
- Avoid exposure
- Wear hypersensitivity bracelet or card

FEMALE
REPRODUCTIVE
SYSTEM

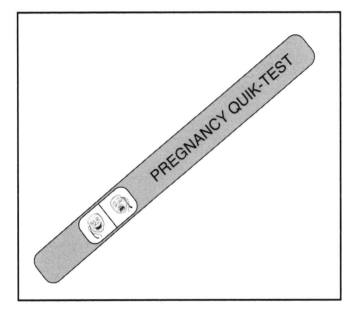

17.1.) MENSTRUAL CYCLE

➤ Days are counted from the <u>first day of the last menstrual period</u>.
➤ Ovulation occurs around day 14 (but is variable because of varying length of the proliferative phases)

proliferative phase	***variable** length (10-20 days, including menstruation)* - ovarian follicle matures - endometrium grows in preparation for implantation
ovulation	***triggered by LH surge*** - may cause "Mittelschmerz" (mid cycle pain) - ovum can be fertilized within 24~36 hours ***
secretory phase	***fixed** length (14 days)* - ruptured follicle transforms to corpus luteum - progesterone from corpus luteum sustains endometrium
menstruation	degeneration of corpus luteum → decline of progesteron → triggers menstruation

 *** *Sperm survives up to 3 days → fertile period is about 5 days!*

CYCLIC CHANGES OF CERVICAL MUCUS:

before and during ovulation	days after ovulation
• thin, watery fluid • stretchy ("Spinnbarkeit") • ferning pattern when dried on a glass slide	• more thick fluid • not stretchy • no ferning pattern

17.2.) CONTRACEPTION

	ESTIMATED PREGNANCY RATE (during first year of "typical use")
no method	85%
withdrawal method	25%
rhythm method	20%
diaphragm	20%
condom	15%
oral contraceptives	6%
IUD	4%
depot-progesterone (Norplant)	< 0.5%

Home pregnancy test:
➤ Measures human chorionic gonadotropin (hCG)
➤ Urine becomes positive 3~4 weeks after conception
            (= 1~2 weeks after missed period)

17.3.) INFERTILITY

ovulatory problems	**abnormal hormone production** - too much androgens or prolactin - lack of gonadotropins (FSH and LH)
pelvic problems	**chronic infections** - salpingitis (gonorrhea, chlamydia) - endometriosis - congenital abnormalities
cervical problems	- abnormal mucus - abnormal Pap smears
male problems	**no sperm** - genetic abnormalities - ductal obstruction - varicocele **few sperm** - maturation arrest - heat *(wear loose pants!)* **abnormal morphology** - infections (mumps) **abnormal motility** - infections (mumps) - immunologic incompatibility

Overall causes of infertility:

50% due to women

30% due to men

20% combination of the two

17.4.) <u>MENSTRUATION</u>

Normal blood loss is 30~50 mL over 4~5 days.

Anovulatory cycles (DUB) are normal for the first 1~2 years after menarche.

polymenorrhea	intervals < 22 days
oligomenorrhea	intervals > 40 days
hypomenorrhea	regular bleeding, decreased amount
metrorrhagia	irregular bleeding, normal amount
menorrhagia	prolonged and excessive bleeding
DUB (dysfunctional uterine bleeding)	excessive uterine bleeding (usually **anovulatory cycles**) [1]

[1] *Estrogen breakthrough bleeding occurs due to lack of progesterone (endometrium keeps building up until it finally breaks down).*

17.5.) PRIMARY AMENORRHEA

= Client never menstruated before

➤ Absence of menses by **age 16** if secondary sexual characteristics are present.
➤ Absence of menses by **age 14** if secondary sexual characteristics are absent.

Turner syndrome	XO (missing X chromosome)
testicular feminization	XY, testosterone receptor defect (genetically male, but fully developed female)
dysgenesis	- absence of tubes, uterus, cervix, upper vagina
Stein-Leventhal (polycystic ovaries)	- **infertility** - **hirsutism** - endometrial hyperplasia
imperforate hymen	- monthly abdominal pain but no menses

TURNER SYNDROME:

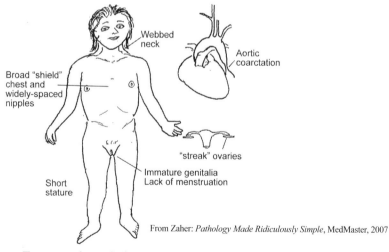

Webbed neck

Aortic coarctation

Broad "shield" chest and widely-spaced nipples

"streak" ovaries

Short stature

Immature genitalia
Lack of menstruation

From Zaher: *Pathology Made Ridiculously Simple*, MedMaster, 2007

Turner syndrome is the most common cause of <u>primary</u> amenorrhea.

17.6.) SECONDARY AMENORRHEA

= Client did have menses previously

➢ Absence of menses for more than 3 cycles.

stress, exercise	- suppressed hypothalamus
anorexia nervosa	- suppressed hypothalamus
post-pill	**- should last no longer than 6 months after discontinuation of pill**
drugs	- antipsychotics - tricyclic antidepressants - benzodiazepines
pituitary failure	**- low FSH and LH**
pituitary neoplasms	**- increased prolactin**

 Pregnancy is the most common cause of <u>secondary</u> amenorrhea.

17.7.) <u>DYSMENORRHEA</u>

ASSESSMENT
◊ Cramping or constant pain in lower abdomen
◊ May radiate to thighs or groin
◊ Lasts 2 - 3 days

IMPLEMENTATION
• Heating pads may help
• Aerobic exercise may help
• Avoid caffeine, alcohol and smoking
MEDICATIONS:
• Analgesics (aspirin, ibuprofen) for mild pain
• Oral contraceptives to suppress ovulation

17.8.) <u>ENDOMETRIOSIS</u>
Presence of endometrial tissue outside of uterine mucosa

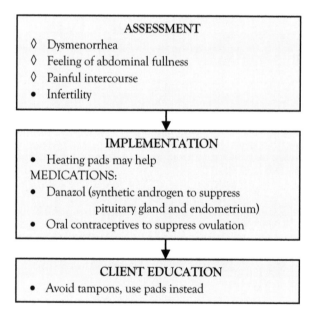

ASSESSMENT
◊ Dysmenorrhea
◊ Feeling of abdominal fullness
◊ Painful intercourse
• Infertility

IMPLEMENTATION
• Heating pads may help
MEDICATIONS:
• Danazol (synthetic androgen to suppress
        pituitary gland and endometrium)
• Oral contraceptives to suppress ovulation

CLIENT EDUCATION
• Avoid tampons, use pads instead

17.9.) <u>PELVIC INFLAMMATORY DISEASE</u>

➤ Often caused by *gonorrhea* or *chlamydia* infection
➤ Risk factors: Multiple sexual partners, IUDs

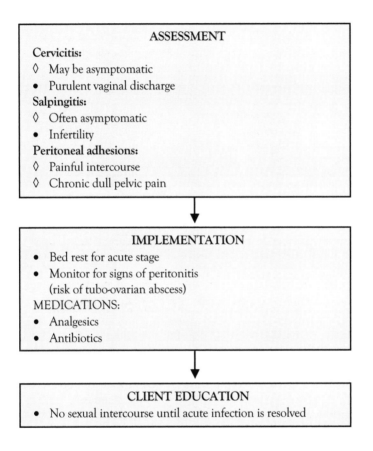

ASSESSMENT

Cervicitis:
◊ May be asymptomatic
• Purulent vaginal discharge
Salpingitis:
◊ Often asymptomatic
• Infertility
Peritoneal adhesions:
◊ Painful intercourse
◊ Chronic dull pelvic pain

IMPLEMENTATION

• Bed rest for acute stage
• Monitor for signs of peritonitis
   (risk of tubo-ovarian abscess)
MEDICATIONS:
• Analgesics
• Antibiotics

CLIENT EDUCATION

• No sexual intercourse until acute infection is resolved

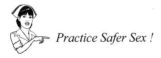

Practice Safer Sex !

17.10.) <u>MENOPAUSE</u>

➢ Ovaries become less sensitive to gonadotropins → estrogen decreases

➢ Premature menopause: client's age < 40 years

➢ Vaginal bleeding due to unopposed estrogen normal for up to 12 months
➢ If vaginal bleeding continues > 12 months: suspect endometrial pathology

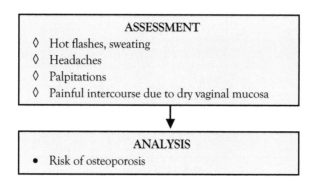

ASSESSMENT
◊ Hot flashes, sweating
◊ Headaches
◊ Palpitations
◊ Painful intercourse due to dry vaginal mucosa

ANALYSIS
• Risk of osteoporosis

ESTROGEN REPLACEMENT THERAPY:

ADVANTAGES	DISADVANTAGES
Relief of menopausal symptoms - eliminates hot flashes - prevents atrophic vagina	**Contraindications** - liver disease - thrombosis, thrombophlebitis
Prevents cardiovascular disease - decreases LDL - increases HDL	**Slightly increased cancer risk** - endometrial carcinoma: 2~8 fold - breast cancer: (controversial)
Prevents osteoporosis - most effective if started early	

17.11.) NIPPLE DISCHARGE

benign epithelial debris	◊ common in middle-aged women with several children • thick, grayish
breast abscess	• thick, purulent
breast cancer	• bloody[1] or watery • sometimes purulent
milky	• phenothiazines, other drugs... • high prolactin levels

[1] *Note however that most bloody discharge is benign!*

17.12.) FIBROCYSTIC CHANGE

Extremely common – not a disease!

FIBROCYSTIC CHANGE	BREAST CANCER
• often bilateral • multiple nodules • menstrual variation • may regress during pregnancy	• often unilateral • single mass • no cyclic variations

17.13.) BREAST CANCER

Most common cancer in women

RISK FACTORS:
➢ Family history
➢ Age of patient
➢ Estrogens

ASSESSMENT
- Palpable breast mass
- Skin dimpling (looks like "orange peel")
- Nipple retraction
- Diagnosis: Mammography, biopsy

IMPLEMENTATION

OPERATIVE:
- **Lumpectomy:** sufficient for early stages
- **Mastectomy:** breast removal, lymph nodes left in place
- **Modified radical mastectomy:** removal of breast and lymph nodes
- **Radical mastectomy:** removal of breast, pectoral muscles and lymph nodes

POSTOPERATIVE:
- Chemotherapy if axillary nodes positive
- Tamoxifen if estrogen receptor positive

CLIENT EDUCATION
- Teach importance of regular self-exam!
- Most cancers develop in outer upper quadrant
- Mammography: every 1-2 years after age 50

17.14.) <u>BREAST SELF-EXAM</u>

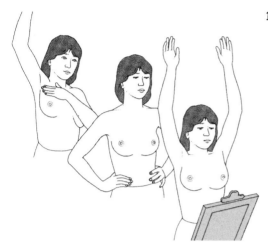

1. **Stand in front of a mirror** and look at each breast to see if there is a lump, a depression, a difference in skin texture or any other change. Be especially alert for any changes in the nipples' appearance. Raise both arms and check for any swelling or dimpling in the skin of your breasts.

2. Lie down with a pillow under your right shoulder and put your right arm behind your head. With the pads of the fingers of your left hand, **make firm circular movements over each quadrant** and feel for any lumps or tenderness. When you reach the upper outer quadrant, continue towards your armpit.

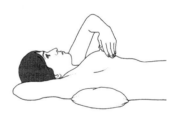

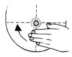

3. Feel your nipple for any change in size and shape. Squeeze your nipple to see if there is **any discharge**.

Adapted from *The American Medical Association Family Medical Guide*, 3rd edition, p. 630, edit
Copyright 1994 by Random House, New York, NY. Used with permission.

17.15.) CERVICAL CANCER

Most cases related to prior infection with papilloma virus!

RISK FACTORS:
- ➤ Multiple sex partners at early age
- ➤ Human papilloma virus (sexually transmitted)
- ➤ Smoking

ASSESSMENT
◊ More common in middle-aged women
◊ Asymptomatic until late stages
PAP SMEAR:
- CIN I or II = cervical dysplasia, increased risk of cancer
- CIN III = carcinoma in situ

IMPLEMENTATION
OPERATIVE:
- **Cryosurgery:** freezing of superficial tissue
- **Conization:** removal of cone shaped slice of cervix
- **Hysterectomy:** removal of uterus
POSTOPERATIVE:
- Monitor for urinary retention
RADIOTHERAPY:
- Isolate client (bed rest required)
- Prevent displacement of radium implant (see 1.9.)

CLIENT EDUCATION
- Pap smear every 2 years for all sexually active women
- Vaccine against papilloma virus is available!

17.16.) <u>OVARIAN CANCER</u>

<u>RISK FACTORS</u>:
- ➢ History of miscarriages or infertility
- ➢ Breast cancer
- ➢ High-fat diet

ASSESSMENT

EARLY:
- ◊ Vague abdominal discomfort
- • Constipation, flatulence

LATE:
- • Palpable abdominal mass
- • Ascites

IMPLEMENTATION

OPERATIVE:
- • **Oophorectomy:** removal of ovaries
    (usually uterus is removed too)

POSTOPERATIVE:
- • Check dressings for excessive bleeding
- • Watch for signs of infection
- • Watch for abdominal distention
- • Chemotherapy or radiotherapy

CLIENT EDUCATION
- • Removal of ovaries in premenopausal woman will induce menopause

---

 Prognosis is poor because of late detection and rapid tumor spread.

17.17.) <u>ENDOMETRIAL CANCER</u>

<u>RISK FACTORS</u>:
➢ Obesity
➢ Nulliparity
➢ Estrogens

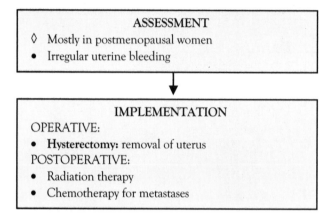

| ASSESSMENT |
| ◊ Mostly in postmenopausal women |
| • Irregular uterine bleeding |

| IMPLEMENTATION |
| OPERATIVE: |
| • **Hysterectomy:** removal of uterus |
| POSTOPERATIVE: |
| • Radiation therapy |
| • Chemotherapy for metastases |

17.18.) <u>UTERINE MYOMAS</u>

➢ Benign tumors of uterine smooth muscle
➢ Regress after menopause

| ASSESSMENT |
| ◊ Small myomas are asymptomatic |
| • Large myomas cause pressure on adjacent organs |
| • Menstrual irregularities |

| IMPLEMENTATION |
| • High-fiber diet to reduce constipation |
| • Surgery only if myomas are large or numerous |

MATERNITY

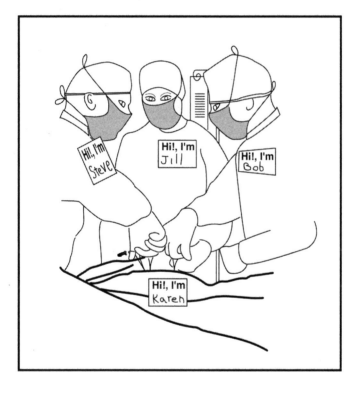

18.1.) PARITY

nulligravida	- client is not and never has been pregnant
primigravida	- client is or has been pregnant - irrespective of pregnancy outcome
nullipara	- client has never completed a pregnancy - may or may not have aborted
primipara	- client has completed one pregnancy (baby > 500g , dead or alive)
multipara	- client has completed two or more pregnancies

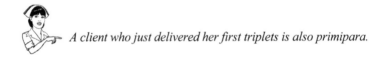

A client who just delivered her first triplets is also primipara.

18.2.) PREGNANCY: SIGNS & SYMPTOMS

presumptive signs	◊ **menses** > 10 days late
	◊ **morning nausea** - occurs at 4~6 weeks of gestation
	◊ **breast changes** - tenderness - enlargement of Montgomery's tubercles
	◊ **quickening** - first perception of fetal movement - occurs at 16~20 weeks
	• **chloasma** - darkening of skin over forehead, bridge of nose and cheekbones
probable signs	• **uterus enlarged** - 12 weeks: above symphysis - 20 weeks: at umbilicus
	• **Hegar's sign** - softening of cervix
	• **Chadwick's sign** - bluish discoloration of cervix
	• **hCG in urine**
certain signs	• **ultrasound identification of fetus** - after 6 weeks
	• **fetal heart tones** - after 17~19 weeks by auscultation

18.3.) PREGNANCY: COMMON PROBLEMS

EARLY PREGNANCY:

nausea, vomiting	- eat crackers before getting up - eat small, frequent meals - vitamin B6 may help
swollen, tender gums	- use soft toothbrush - maintain good nutrition
breast tenderness	- wear supportive bra

LATE PREGNANCY:

heartburn	- avoid fatty, spicy meals - sit upright 30 minutes after meal
constipation	- increase fluid and fiber intake - walking
backache	- wear low-heeled shoes
ankle edema, varicose veins	- elevate legs frequently - avoid crossing legs - wear supportive stocking

18.4.) PREGNANCY: SIGNS OF DANGER

persistent vomiting	hyperemesis gravidarum
edema of legs and face, hypertension	preeclampsia
abdominal pain	premature labor abruptio placentae
bleeding from vagina	abruptio placentae placenta previa "bloody show"
leak of clear fluid from vagina	premature rupture of membranes
absence of fetal movements	fetal death

18.5.) <u>FIRST TRIMESTER</u>

ASSESSMENT
- Presumptive and probable signs
- Bleeding is common
  (50% result in spontaneous abortion, 50% continue normally)

ANALYSIS
- Presence of risk factors?

IMPLEMENTATION
- History: First day of last menstrual period?
- Childhood diseases: measles, rubella?
- Immunizations?
- Past pregnancies?
- Blood type and Rhesus factor?
- Drug abuse?
ULTRASOUND:
- To confirm and date pregnancy

CLIENT EDUCATION
- Increase caloric intake by 300 kcal/day
- Increase protein intake
- Expect weight gain of 3-4 lb. during 1st trimester
- Vitamin supplementation, especially folic acid!

Dr. Nägele's rule:
"9 month plus 7 days from beginning of LMP."
Dr. Carl's rule:
"Rarely do they come on the day expected."

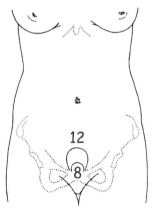

18.6.) <u>SECOND TRIMESTER</u>

ASSESSMENT
- ◊ Client feels quickening (fetal movements)
- Fundus at level of umbilicus at 20 weeks
- Nausea and vomiting have ceased
- Fetal heart rate 120-160 per minute
- Bleeding → suspect low-lying placenta

ANALYSIS
- Risk factors for preeclampsia?
- Risk factors for preterm delivery?

CLIENT EDUCATION
- Expect additional weight gain of 1 lb. per week
- Wear low-heeled shoes
- Avoid high-impact aerobics
- Avoid hot tubs and saunas
- Recommend Lamaze classes

<u>RISK FACTORS FOR
PRETERM LABOR</u>:
- ➤ Multiple gestation
- ➤ History of abortions
- ➤ Client younger than 15 years
- ➤ Client older than 35 years
- ➤ Poor nutrition
- ➤ Alcohol or drug use
- ➤ Smoking

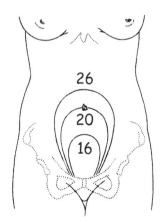

From *Danforth's obstetrics and gynecology*, 7th edition, p. 77, edited by J.R. Scott et al.
Copyright 1994 by Lippincott-Raven Publishers, Philadelphia, PA. Used with permission.

18.7.) __THIRD TRIMESTER__

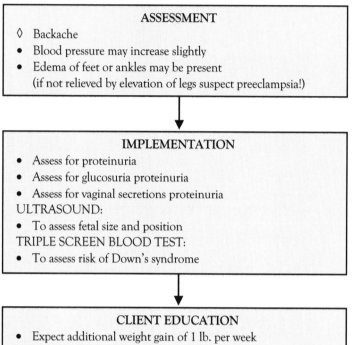

ASSESSMENT
◊ Backache
• Blood pressure may increase slightly
• Edema of feet or ankles may be present
  (if not relieved by elevation of legs suspect preeclampsia!)

↓

IMPLEMENTATION
• Assess for proteinuria
• Assess for glucosuria proteinuria
• Assess for vaginal secretions proteinuria
ULTRASOUND:
• To assess fetal size and position
TRIPLE SCREEN BLOOD TEST:
• To assess risk of Down's syndrome

↓

CLIENT EDUCATION
• Expect additional weight gain of 1 lb. per week
• Teach "true" and "false" signs of labor (see 18.12)
• Use good body mechanics
• Rest with legs elevated

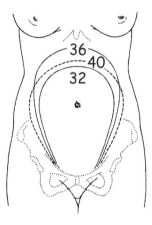

AMNIOCENTESIS:
➢ Aspiration of fluid from uterine cavity
➢ To asses fetal abnormalities
➢ To assess fetal lung maturity
➢ Significant risk of fetal loss!

18.8.) PREECLAMPSIA

➢ **High risk groups:** African Americans and young primipara.

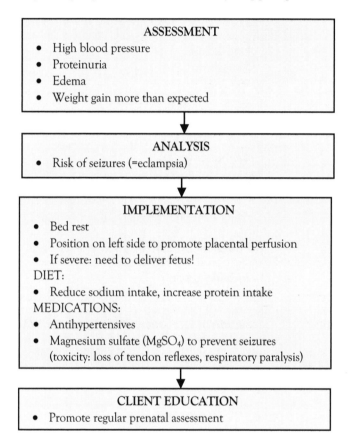

ASSESSMENT
- High blood pressure
- Proteinuria
- Edema
- Weight gain more than expected

ANALYSIS
- Risk of seizures (=eclampsia)

IMPLEMENTATION
- Bed rest
- Position on left side to promote placental perfusion
- If severe: need to deliver fetus!

DIET:
- Reduce sodium intake, increase protein intake

MEDICATIONS:
- Antihypertensives
- Magnesium sulfate ($MgSO_4$) to prevent seizures
  (toxicity: loss of tendon reflexes, respiratory paralysis)

CLIENT EDUCATION
- Promote regular prenatal assessment

Have calcium gluconate ready to counteract overdose of $MgSO_4$!

18.9.) THE FETUS

fetal lie	*long axis of fetus in relation to long axis of uterus* - longitudinal - transverse - oblique

fetal presentation	*portion of fetus that can be felt through cervix*
	
	- **cephalic:** vertex
	             face
	             brow
	
	- **frank breech** (thighs are flexed, legs are extended)
	
	- **complete breech** (thighs are flexed, legs are flexed)
	
	- **footling breech**

fetal position	*relation of fetal occiput to maternal birth canal*

Normal position
(head first – occiput anterior)

Frank Breech presentation

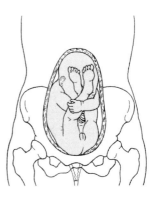

Full Breech presentation

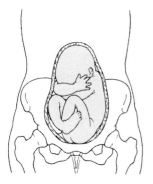

Footling Breech presentation

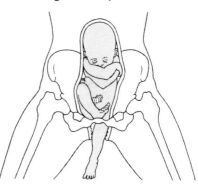

From *The Source Book of Medical Illustration*, 2nd edition, pp. 294-9, edited by P. Cull.
Copyright 1991 by Parthenon Publishing Group Limited, Lancaster, England.

18.10.) FETAL EVALUATION

nonstress test [1]	- 3 or more fetal movements in 30 min - heart rate accelerations > 15 beats/min
oxytocin stress test [2]	- no late decelerations - (early decelerations are o.k.)

[1] *normal fetal activity should result in heart rate increases*
[2] *tests ability of fetus to withstand uterine contractions*

18.11.) FETAL HEART RATE

normal	- **good variability** (120 to 160 beats/min)
decreased variability	- CNS depression (often due to medications)
early decelerations	- not a/w poor fetal outcome - not caused by hypoxemia
late decelerations	- **fetal hypoxemia and distress** - a/w preeclampsia, maternal hypotension, excessive uterine contractions

18.12.) ASSESSMENT: LABOR

	"TRUE LABOR"	"FALSE LABOR"
intervals	regular	irregular
contractions	intensity increases gradually	intensity constant
walking	increases contractions	decreases contractions
sedation	does not affect contractions	stops contractions

1st stage	- lasts about 12 hours (primipara) - cervix effacement and dilation - **latent phase**: slow dilation of cervix - **active phase**: rapid dilation of cervix
2nd stage	- lasts about 1 hour (primipara) - delivery of infant
3rd stage	- within 30 minutes - delivery of placenta

18.13.) <u>LABOR: FIRST STAGE</u>

➢ Begins with "true" contractions, ends with complete dilation of cervix.

<u>BLEEDING</u>:

bloody show	- mixed with mucus
placenta previa	- heavy, painless bleeding
abruptio placentae	- none or heavy bleeding - continuous abdominal pain
uterus rupture	- sudden cessation of uterine contractions - disappearance of fetal heart tones

---

IMPLEMENTATION

FETUS:
- Determine fetal position
- Monitor fetal heart rate: variability and decelerations

MOTHER:
- Assess vital signs every 60 minutes
- Assess contractions: frequency, duration, intensity
- Nitrazine test to determine whether membranes are ruptured
- Monitor and chart cervix dilation and effacement

- Encourage client to void every 2 hours
- Discourage use of perineal pads: moist environment → risk of infection
- Discourage pushing before cervical dilation is complete
- Only clear liquids and ice chips are allowed!

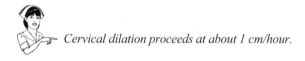

Cervical dilation proceeds at about 1 cm/hour.

18.14.) LABOR: SECOND STAGE

➢ Ends with delivery of baby.

IMPLEMENTATION
- Assess vital signs every 15 minutes
- Monitor fetal heart rate: variability and decelerations
- Provide physical comfort, massages
- Support client's body and extremities during pushing

CLIENT EDUCATION
- Breathe in through nose, out through mouth
- Push only during contractions

FETAL STAGE:
➢   -3, -2, -1   cm above ischial spines
➢   0   at level of ischial spines
➢   +1, +2, +3   cm below ischial spines

18.15.) LABOR: THIRD STAGE

➢ Ends with delivery of placenta.

IMPLEMENTATION
- Delivery of placenta should occur within 30min. of birth
- Don't pull at umbilical cord!
- Evaluate placenta for completeness
- Massage uterine fundus

18.16.) SPONTANEOUS ABORTION

threatened abortion	- bleeding - uterine cramping - **no cervical dilation**
inevitable abortion	- bleeding - uterine cramping - **ruptured membranes** - **cervix dilated**
incomplete abortion	- **retained placental tissue**
early abortion	- very common [1] - often unnoticed - usually due to chromosomal abnormalities
missed abortion	- **death of fetus or embryo** - no labor or passage of tissue
habitual abortion	- three or more spontaneous abortions

[1] *about 50% of all conceptions (fertilized eggs) are lost spontaneously*

CAUSES OF HABITUAL ABORTION:
➤ Chromosomal abnormalities
➤ Cervical incompetence
➤ Infections
➤ Hormonal dysfunction

18.17.) <u>PREMATURE LABOR</u>
Before completing 37 weeks of gestation

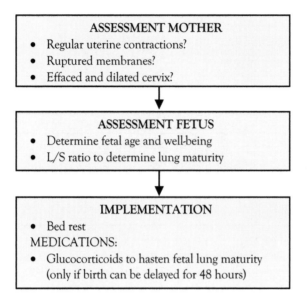

ASSESSMENT MOTHER
- Regular uterine contractions?
- Ruptured membranes?
- Effaced and dilated cervix?

ASSESSMENT FETUS
- Determine fetal age and well-being
- L/S ratio to determine lung maturity

IMPLEMENTATION
- Bed rest

MEDICATIONS:
- Glucocorticoids to hasten fetal lung maturity (only if birth can be delayed for 48 hours)

18.18.) <u>CESAREAN SECTION</u>

In the past, if a client had a C-section all future births would need to be delivered by C-section because of the high risk of uterine rupture. Nowadays, if the previous C-section was done with a low transverse incision, subsequent vaginal births are possible.

<u>INDICATIONS</u>:
- ➤ Frank breech presentation
- ➤ Fetal distress
- ➤ Prolapsed cord
- ➤ Abruptio placentae
- ➤ Active genital herpes

18.19.) ABRUPTIO PLACENTAE

ASSESSMENT
◊ Continuous abdominal pain
• Heavy bleeding (but may be concealed!)
• Sustained uterine contraction
• Fetal distress
• DIC

IMPLEMENTATION
• Treat shock: IV fluids, oxygen
• Left lateral position to enhance placental perfusion
• Monitor coagulation status
• Prepare for immediate C section

18.20.) PROLAPSED CORD

RISK FACTORS:
➤ Breech presentation
➤ Multiple pregnancy
➤ Prematurity

ASSESSMENT
• Fetal hypoxia
• Irregular fetal heart rate
• Umbilical cord can be seen or felt (not always!)

IMPLEMENTATION
• Monitor fetal heart rate continuously
• Elevate fetal presenting part to relieve pressure
• Do not push cord back into uterus!
• Prepare for immediate C-section

18.21.) <u>POSTPARTUM HEMORRHAGE</u>

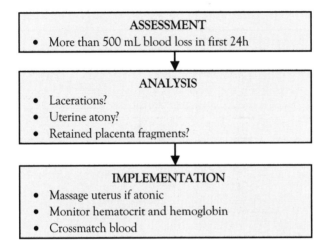

ASSESSMENT
- More than 500 mL blood loss in first 24h

ANALYSIS
- Lacerations?
- Uterine atony?
- Retained placenta fragments?

IMPLEMENTATION
- Massage uterus if atonic
- Monitor hematocrit and hemoglobin
- Crossmatch blood

18.22.) <u>PUERPERAL INFECTION</u>

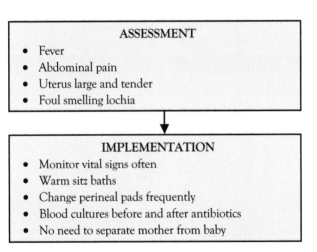

ASSESSMENT
- Fever
- Abdominal pain
- Uterus large and tender
- Foul smelling lochia

IMPLEMENTATION
- Monitor vital signs often
- Warm sitz baths
- Change perineal pads frequently
- Blood cultures before and after antibiotics
- No need to separate mother from baby

Dr. Semmelweiss' great advice: **"Always wash your hands!"**

18.23.) <u>MASTITIS</u>

Inflammation → obstruction of ducts → milk stasis

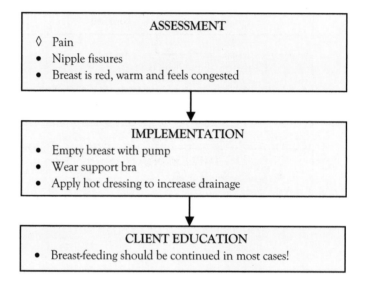

ASSESSMENT
◊ Pain
- Nipple fissures
- Breast is red, warm and feels congested

IMPLEMENTATION
- Empty breast with pump
- Wear support bra
- Apply hot dressing to increase drainage

CLIENT EDUCATION
- Breast-feeding should be continued in most cases!

HIV positive clients should not breast-feed their infants because of high risk transmitting the HIV virus!

GROWTH
&
DEVELOPMENT

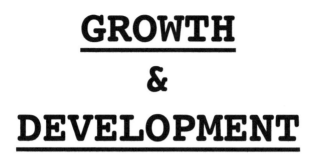

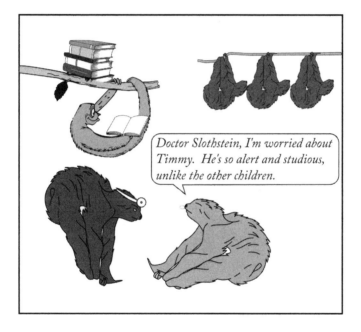

19.1.) <u>NUTRITION</u>

breast milk	• **compared to cow milk:** - more fat - more carbohydrates - both lack vitamin D
supplementation	• **iron** - start supplementation at age 4~6 months (earlier in preterm infants) • **fluoride** - for all breast fed infants - or if Fl⁻ content of drinking water is poor • **Ca^{2+}, vitamin D** - for breast fed infants at risk (little sunlight etc.) • **vitamin B12** - for breast fed infants if mother is vegetarian
commercial formulas	• **cow milk based** (with added whey protein) • **soy protein formulas** - hypoallergenic - useful after diarrhea (transient lactase deficiency)

 Human milk is best for humans, cow milk is best for calves.

19.2.) <u>MOTOR DEVELOPMENT</u>

chin up	1 month
chest up	2 month
knee push and "swim"	6 month
sits alone / stands with help	7 month
crawls on stomach	8 month
stands holding on furniture	10 month
walks when led	11 month
stands alone	14 month
walks alone	15 month

2 months   7 months   8 months   15 months

<u>AT THE PLAYGROUND</u>:
- Stranger anxiety: 0 ~ 1 years
- Separation anxiety: 1 ~ 3 years
- Parallel play: 2 ~ 3 years
- Group play: 3 ~ 4 years

19.3.) PSYCHOLOGICAL DEVELOPMENT

years	Erikson	Freud	Piaget
0 ~ 1.5	trust vs. mistrust	oral (trust & dependence)	sensorimotor
1.5 ~ 3	autonomy vs. shame	anal (holding vs. letting out)	preoperational
3 ~ 6	initiative vs. guilt	phallic (Oedipus complex)	"
6 ~ 11	industry vs. inferiority	latency	concrete operational
11 ~ 20	identity vs. role confusion	genital	formal operational
20 ~ 25	intimacy vs. isolation		
25 ~ 50	generativity vs. stagnation		
50 ~ ?	integrity vs. despair		

19.4.) IQ TESTS

DEVIATION TESTS	TESTS OF MENTAL AGE
mean: 100 **standard deviation:** 15	IQ = mental age / biological age
EXAMPLE:	EXAMPLE:
- IQ 85 is one standard deviation below the average	a 16-year old performs at the level of a 14-year old → IQ = 14/16 = 88
- IQ 70 is two standard deviations below the average	

➤ 68% of people are within ± 1 standard deviation
➤ 95% of people are within ± 2 standard deviations

DEGREES OF MENTAL RETARDATION:

IQ 55 ~ 70 (mild)	mentally handicapped but educable
IQ 40 ~ 55 (moderate)	trainable for personal hygiene
IQ 25 ~ 40 (severe)	custodial
IQ < 25 (profound)	custodial

AUTISM:
- Impaired social interaction
- Impaired communication
- Stereotypic behavior
- IQ may be normal (but difficult to test)

297

19.5.) FAILURE TO THRIVE

= slow growth and mental development in first 3 years of life

---

ASSESSMENT
- Growth below 3rd percentile
  (2 standard deviations below average)
- Apathy, weakness, irritability
- Lack of social responses (eye contact, smiles)

↓

ANALYSIS

PHYSIOLOGIC INTEGRITY:
- Inborn errors of metabolism?
- Endocrine function?
- Neurological dysfunction?

SAFE, EFFECTIVE CARE ENVIRONMENT:
- Caring family?
- Alcohol or drug abuse?
- Child abuse?

↓

IMPLEMENTATION
- Provide sensory stimulation:
  - cuddling, rocking, talking
  - colorful toys
- Observe parent-child interaction
- Arrange for alternative placement of child if necessary

↓

CLIENT EDUCATION
- Develop home-care plan with parents
- Referral for financial or mental health assistance

19.6.) CHILD ABUSE

A) FORMS OF ABUSE:

➢ Physical
➢ Emotional
➢ Sexual
➢ Neglect

B) SIGNS & SYMPTOMS:

PERHAPS ACCIDENTAL	MORE LIKELY INTENTIONAL
• splash marks • injuries to front • foot soles spared	• clearly demarcated areas, no splash • injuries to back • foot soles involved
	◊ history of multiple injuries • retinal hemorrhage ("shaken baby")

 Involve Department of Social Services early!

THE NEONATE

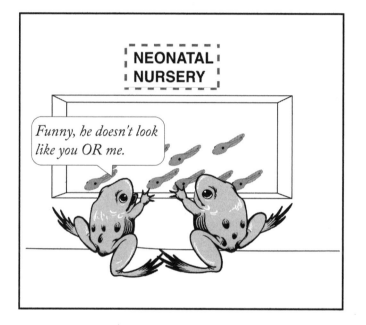

20.1.) BIRTH TRAUMA

subdural hemorrhage	- **mechanical trauma, forceps** - more common in large infants
cephalhematoma	- subperiosteal hemorrhage - **limited to area of affected bone**
caput succedaneum	- diffuse edema of scalp soft tissue - **not limited to area of bones**
Erb-Duchenne paralysis [1]	**"waiter's tip" position:** - forearm extended and internally rotated - wrist flexed
Klumpke paralysis [2]	- distal arm paralysis - wrist drop
amnion band syndrome	- loss of a digit or limb due to constriction - a/w early rupture of membranes

[1] *injury to superior brachial plexus*
[2] *injury to inferior brachial plexus*

20.2.) APGAR SCORE

	0	1	2
A - Appearance	blue, pale	acrocyanosis	pink
P - Pulse rate	none	< 100/min	> 100/min
G - Grimace	absent	grimace	cough or sneeze
A - Activity	limp muscles	some flexion	active motion
R - Respiration	none	slow, irregular	good, crying

7 or above is good.
Apgar score does not indicate long-term prognosis.

20.3.) VITAL SIGNS (NEWBORN)

NORMAL RANGES:

heart rate	120 - 140 / minute
respirations	30 - 50 / minute
blood pressure	systolic ~70, diastolic ~45 mmHg

20.4.) <u>REFLEXES</u>

sucking reflex **palmar grasp reflex**	- weak in premature infants - fully developed after 36 weeks of gestation

tonic neck reflex	- turn face to one side (supine position):
	  arms and leg on face side will extend
	
	- indicates neurological dysfunction if
	  constantly present

automatic walking	- full-term newborns at 40 weeks tend to
	  "walk" in heel-toe progression
	
	- preterm infants at 40 weeks tend to "walk"
	  in toe-heel progression

Babinski reflex	**- normal up to 2 years of age** - firmly stroke lateral sole of feet - dorsiflexion of great toe, fanning of other toes
Moro reflex "startle reflex"	**- normal up to 6 months of age**

From *The Lippincott Manual of Nursing Practice*, 6th edition, p. 1097, edited by S.M. Nettina
Copyright 1996 by Lippincott-Raven Publishers, Philadelphia, PA. Used with permission.

20.5.) SMALL & LARGE INFANTS

SMALL FOR GESTATIONAL AGE	LARGE FOR GESTATIONAL AGE
2 SD below expected (smaller than 97% of infants)	**2 SD above expected (larger than 97% of infants)**
- chromosomal abnormalities - intrauterine infections (viruses) - alcohol, drug abuse - maternal hypertension - placenta insufficiency	- diabetic mother
• Maintain airways and temperature • Observe for respiratory distress	• Maintain airways and temperature • Monitor glucose levels (risk of hypoglycemia if mother diabetic)

SD = standard deviation

 Low birth weight infant: *< 2,500 g at birth (can be SGA, normal or LGA)*

> ### Problems of infants of diabetic mothers:
> ➤ Birth trauma
> ➤ Hypoglycemia
> ➤ Respiratory distress syndrome

20.6.) PREMATURITY

= born before completing 37 weeks, irrespective of birth weight

---

ASSESSMENT

- Skin is thin and red, appears opaque with visible veins
- Lanugo hair on back and face
- Absent skin creases on palms and soles
- Females: prominent clitoris
- Males: underdeveloped scrotum
- Weak reflexes (grasping, sucking, swallowing)

IMPLEMENTATION

- Provide external warmth and humidity
  (infant is unable to maintain body temperature)
- Gavage feeding
- Infection control procedures
- Frequent Assessment of physiological integrity:
  - **Respiration**: watch rate, rhythm, secretions, nasal flaring
  - **Heart**: watch rate, rhythm and murmurs
  - **GI tract**: watch for abdominal distention, bowel sounds
  - **Nervous system**: check reflexes and pupils

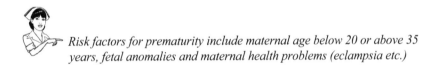

Risk factors for prematurity include maternal age below 20 or above 35 years, fetal anomalies and maternal health problems (eclampsia etc.)

20.7.) POSTMATURITY

= born after 42 weeks, irrespective of birth weight

ASSESSMENT

- Dry, wrinkled skin
- Long nails
- Loss of subcutaneous fat
- Meconium staining

20.8.) RESPIRATORY DISTRESS SYNDROME

Hyaline membrane disease - due to lung immaturity

risk factors	- male sex - premature birth - second born twin - perinatal asphyxia - maternal diabetes
signs & symptoms	• nasal flaring (inspiratory) • grunting (expiratory) • tachypnea • cyanosis • fluid filled alveoli
complications	- pneumonia - pneumothorax **oxygen toxicity:** - bronchopulmonary dysplasia - retinopathy

ANALYSIS
• Impaired gas exchange

IMPLEMENTATION
• Keep head aligned with body, neck slightly extended
• Monitor oxygen administration (PEEP)
• Remove airway secretions frequently
  (gag reflex is weak!)
MEDICATIONS:
• Surfactant via endotracheal tube

20.9.) NEONATAL JAUNDICE

physiologic jaundice	- **3 to 5 days postnatal** - due to increased bilirubin from breakdown of fetal red blood cells - relatively immature liver unable to conjugate large amounts of bilirubin
breast milk jaundice	- **2 to 3 weeks after birth** - due to increased bilirubin absorption - *consider brief interruption of breast feeding (but usually not necessary)*
hemolysis	- Rh, ABO incompatibility - RBC abnormalities
kernicterus	- **if unconjugated bilirubin > 20 mg/dL** - staining of basal ganglia • lethargy, hypotonia, encephalopathy

---

IMPLEMENTATION

PHOTOTHERAPY:
• Shield infant's eyes
• Avoid oily lotions on skin
• Turn frequently to expose all skin surfaces
• Monitor temperature and assess for dehydration every 2 hours
EXCHANGE TRANSFUSIONS:
• Parental consent!
• Cross-match blood (double-check!)
• Monitor vital signs every 5 minutes
• Keep record of amounts transfused

20.10.) <u>NEONATAL SEPSIS</u>

Invasive bacterial infection → bacteria and toxins enter blood stream
(onset 3 days to 4 weeks after birth)

ASSESSMENT

- "Non-specific" signs
- Irritability, lethargy
- Altered vital signs: tachypnea, tachycardia, hypotension
- Leukocytosis on CBC

IMPLEMENTATION

- Provide external warmth
  (keep temperature around 98.8°F)
- Monitor vital signs frequently
- Administer and monitor IV infusions
- Assess hydration

MEDICATIONS:

- Broad-spectrum antibiotics

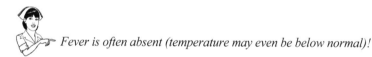 *Fever is often absent (temperature may even be below normal)!*

20.11.) TERATOGENS

= substances that interferes with prenatal development

	DEVELOPMENTAL DEFECTS
alcohol	• **mental retardation** • small eyes • flat nose • broad upper lip
retinoids	• **severe CNS abnormalities** • heart defects • ear malformation (small or absent)
diphenylhydantoin	• **short distal phalanges** • **small finger and toe nails** • flat nasal bridge • cleft lip/palate
warfarin	• **chondrodysplasia** • small head • flat nose
thalidomide	• absence of portion of limbs (hands or feet directly attached to trunk)

Some common drugs that should <u>NOT</u> be given to pregnant women:

➢ Sulfonylureas
➢ Warfarin
➢ Quinine
➢ Tetracyclines

➢ Ibuprofen
➢ Indomethacin
➢ Thiazides
➢ Steroids

20.12.) <u>MULTIFACTORIAL BIRTH DEFECTS</u>

cleft lip / cleft palate	- recurrence risk 2~5%
anencephaly **spina bifida**	- increased risk in women with folate deficiency (1mg/d during pregnancy recommended)
congenital heart defects	- no specific cause - common component of many syndromes

20.13.) HEART DEFECTS: WHAT TO EXPECT

➤ **Acyanotic defects:** Left to right shunt (arterial blood moves to right heart)

Atrial Septal Defect
- If large, consider surgical correction (best done at ages 2~4 years)
- If untreated: shunt reversal and heart failure common in third or fourth decade

Ventricular Septal Defect
- If small expect spontaneous closure
- Elective surgery at 2~4 years

Patent Ductus Arteriosus
- Indomethacin facilitates spontaneous closure
- Elective surgery at 1~2 years

➤ **Cyanotic defects:** Right to left shunt (venous blood enters systemic circulation)

Fallot's Tetralogy
- Most common <u>cyanotic</u> congenital heart defect
- Total correction required

Transposition of the Great Arteries
- Newborn: palliative enlargement of atrial septal defect
- Total correction required (high surgical mortality)

A) <u>Transposition of Great Arteries</u>

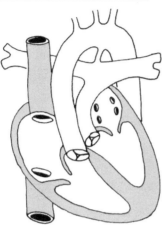

From Goldberg: *Clinical Anatomy Made Ridiculously Simple*, MedMaster, 2007

B) <u>Tetralogy of Fallot</u>

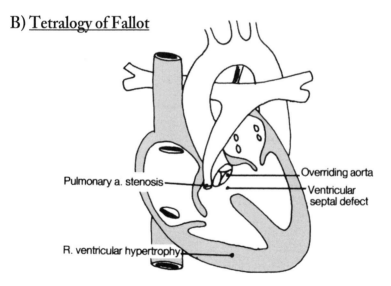

From Goldberg: *Clinical Anatomy Made Ridiculously Simple*, MedMaster, 2007

20.14.) <u>CEREBRAL PALSY</u>

➤ Preventive measures: improve prenatal care and obstetric management!

ASSESSMENT
- Spasticity (hypertonicity of muscles)
- Athetosis (slow, involuntary writhing movements)
- Drooling, impaired speech
- Persistent primitive reflexes

↓

ANALYSIS
- Impaired physical mobility
- Risk of seizures
- Risk of injuries

↓

IMPLEMENTATION
- Safe environment: side rails on bed, padding
- Restrain when in chair to prevent falls
- Provide helmet if prone to falls
- Have child assist in care as much as possible (encourage self-dressing etc.)
- Speech therapy

↓

CLIENT EDUCATION
- Teach parents how to correctly use braces and splints
- Help parents with physical therapy regimen

20.15.) <u>DOWN'S SYNDROME</u>
= trisomy 21 (extra chromosome usually of maternal origin)

ASSESSMENT
- Epicanthal folds ("mongoloid look")
- Eyes slant upward and outward
- Flat nasal bridge ("saddle nose")
- Hypotonic muscles ("floppy infant")
- Horizontal palmar crease
- Protruding tongue
- Increased incidence of congenital cardiac defects

ANALYSIS
- Mental retardation (mild to moderate)

IMPLEMENTATION
- Help family to accept
- Help family to identify short- and long-term goals
- Promote self-help, social skills and independence:
  (speech, physical and occupational therapy)

CLIENT EDUCATION
- Genetic counseling
- Recurrence risk usually 1%
  (much higher if due to abnormal parental karyotype)

Increased risk if mother >30 years old. Risk can be estimated using the "triple screen" blood test. If positive, consider amniocentesis.

20.16.) <u>ESOPHAGEAL ATRESIA</u>

Esophagus often has connection (fistula) to trachea → high risk of aspiration

---

ASSESSMENT
- Excessive salivation and drooling
- 3 Cs: Coughing, Choking, Cyanosis (during feeding)
- Diagnosis: catheter probe or radiographic

↓

IMPLEMENTATION
- Elevate head of bed to prevent esophageal reflux into lung
- Aspirate secretions from blind pouch
  (have suction available at all times!)
- Feed via gastrostomy tube

POSTOPERATIVE:
- Observe closely for choking
- Avoid hyperextension of neck to protect suture line
- Percussion and postural drainage

20.17.) <u>HYPERTROPHIC PYLORIC STENOSIS</u>

ASSESSMENT
- Projectile vomiting shortly after meals
- Weight loss, dehydration
- Metabolic alkalosis (loss of acid)
- Olive-shaped mass palpable in right upper quadrant

↓

IMPLEMENTATION
- Monitor intake / output
- Feed slowly, hold infant semi-upright
- Place on right side after feeding, head of mattress elevated

SURGERY:
- Pyloromyotomy = widening of pylorus
- Assure family that outcome is usually excellent

20.18.) <u>INTUSSUSCEPTION</u>

Invagination (slipping) of sections of intestine into one another

---

ASSESSMENT
- ◊ Sudden colicky abdominal pain
- • Infant draws knees towards chest
- • Acute abdomen (tender and hard)
- • Currant-jelly stools (blood and mucus)

↓

IMPLEMENTATION
- • Monitor stools:
  (brown stool may indicate reduction of intussusception)
- • Monitor vital signs
- • NPO, maintain patency of nasogastric tube
- • Prepare for emergency surgery

20.19.) <u>HIRSCHSPRUNG'S DISEASE</u>

Absence of ganglion cells → spastic, contracted segment of colon
Colon in front of this segment becomes widely distended (megacolon).

ASSESSMENT
- • Absence of meconium stool in newborns
- • Bile-stained vomiting
- • Distended abdomen
- • Palpable fecal masses

↓

IMPLEMENTATION
- • Record time, form and amount of feces
- • Daily enemas may be necessary
POSTOPERATIVE:
- • Avoid taking temperature rectally
- • Monitor stool consistency
- • Colostomy care
- • Explain parents that colostomy is only temporary
  (correction usually done after age of 6 months)

20.20.) <u>CONGENITAL HIP DYSPLASIA</u>
Maldeveloped hip/femur head joint

ASSESSMENT
- Unequal gluteal folds (higher on affected side)
- Leg appears shorter (on affected side)
- Limited hip abduction on affected side
- **Ortolani sign:** clicking sound occurs if femur head pops out of acetabulum during careful abduction and rotation of hip joint

- If bilateral and untreated: marked lordosis, waddling gait

IMPLEMENTATION
- Teach family how to use and maintain corrective device (abduction brace)

ORTOLANI SIGN:

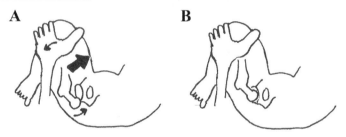

From Tétreault &Ouellette: *Orthopedics Made Ridiculously Simple*, MedMaster, 2009

A: The examiner exerts an upward force (thick black arrow) with a twist (thin black arrow) to reduce the dislocated hip.

B: The Ortolani sign is positive when the hip reduces with this maneuver. A negative Ortolani sign implies that the hip is in a fixed dislocation position.

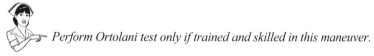

Perform Ortolani test only if trained and skilled in this maneuver.

318

INFANTS
&
TODDLERS

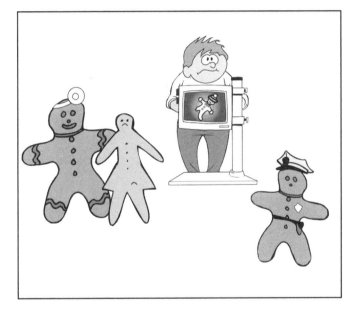

21.1.) THE ILL CHILD

toddler (1~3 yrs)	separation anxiety
preschool (3~6 yrs)	fear of bodily harm fear of mutilation fear of castration
school-age (6~12 yrs)	fear about separation from peers fear about "fitting in"
adolescent (12~18 yrs)	fear of loss of independence fear of loss of privacy

21.2.) PROPER POSITION

PRONE:
➤ Preterm infants with respiratory distress or infants with gastroesophageal reflux do better sleeping in prone position.

SUPINE:
➤ All other infants should be placed in supine or lateral position.
  (significantly reduces risk of *Sudden Infant Death Syndrome*.)

21.3.) <u>DIAPER DERMATITIS</u>

ASSESSMENT
- If in folds: due to heat, moisture or seborrheic dermatitis
- If folds are spared: due to contact dermatitis
- If perianal: due to mechanical or chemical irritation
- Tiny reddish vesicles = "heat rash"

CLIENT EDUCATION
- Change diaper as soon as wet
- Change at least once per night
- Use diapers with moisture absorbent gel
- Avoid occlusive diaper coverings: plastic pants etc.
- Avoid use of powders (especially cornstarch)

21.4.) <u>CRYPTORCHIDISM</u>
= undescended testes (one or both)

ASSESSMENT
◊ Usually asymptomatic
- Empty scrotum
- Testes may be palpable in inguinal canal

CLIENT EDUCATION
IF NOT CORRECTED BY SURGERY:
- Increased risk for testicular cancer
- Decreased or absent sperm production → reduced fertility
- Androgen production is still o.k. → expect normal puberty

Keep observing: 80% of undescended testes will be in the scrotum by age of 1 year. If still undescended, surgery should be done between ages 1 and 3.

21.5.) INFECTIOUS DISEASES OF CHILDHOOD

	SIGNS & SYMPTOMS	NURSING CARE & TREATMENT
MEASLES (rubeola)	**- 3 to 5 days prodrome (cough, running nose, conjunctivitis)** - followed by Koplik's spots - then maculopapular rash: neck → face → arms → trunk	• dim light if child is photophobic • avoid salicylates in infants (better to use acetaminophen)
GERMAN MEASLES (rubella)	**- mild prodrome, tender lymph nodes** - maculopapular rash, 3 day fever rash: neck → face → arms → trunk	• prevent contact with pregnant women!
ROSEOLA (exanthema subitum)	- acute high fever **- maculopapular rash starts as fever falls** - rash begins on trunk	• bed rest during fever • antipyretic

	SIGNS & SYMPTOMS	NURSING CARE & TREATMENT

CHICKENPOX
(varicella)
	- mild prodrome, anorexia
	
	- **papules, vesicles and crusts**
	- begin on trunk → face, extremities
	- lesions at different stages of healing
		• prevent scratching, trim nails
		  (risk of scars or secondary infections)
		• soothing lotion for pruritic area
		• patients with herpes zoster can transmit
		  virus to persons who never had chickenpox

FIFTH DISEASE (erythema infectiosum)	- no prodrome, no fever - sudden bright rash **"slapped cheeks"** - followed by maculopapular rash on trunk and extremities	• no treatment needed

SCARLET FEVER	- Strep. throat plus rash
	  (toxin producing strands of Streptococci)
	- rapid onset fever, headache, vomiting
	
	- **"sand paper" rash**
	- **starts at time of fever**
	- **spares the face**
	- strawberry tongue
		• full course of penicillin
		  (to prevent later complications of
		  streptococcal infection)
		• teach family importance to complete
		  antibiotic treatment

323

	SIGNS & SYMPTOMS	NURSING CARE & TREATMENT
MUMPS	- 24h prodromal stage: fever, headache - **parotid enlargement** within 3 days	• soft and bland food to reduce salivation • local heat or cold may provide relief • orchitis: analgesics and scrotal support
PERTUSSIS	- highly contagious - **catarrhal stage:** coryza, sneezing - **paroxysmal stage:** bursts of coughing high pitched sound on inspiration (whoop) cyanosis, vomiting after attack	• Erythromycin for patient and all household contacts • nutritional support • encourage fluid intake • keep air well humid, dust-free • cough suppressants are of little benefit
INFECTIOUS MONONUCLEOSIS	- headache, malaise, fever - sore throat - splenomegaly - macular eruption (trunk)	• gargles, analgesics for throat • normal activity as tolerated (avoid contact sports → spleen rupture) • Diagnosis: Monospot test

21.6.) <u>INCUBATION PERIODS</u>

	INCUBATION	PATIENT CAN INFECT OTHERS
easles	1 week	7 days before until 5 days after rash onset
rman measles	2 ~ 3 weeks	7 days before until 5 days after rash onset
ickenpox	2 ~ 3 weeks	from onset of fever until last vesicle is dry
umps	2 ~ 3 weeks	7 days before until 9 days after swelling onset
rtussis	1 week	from catarrhal stage until cough subsides
arlet fever	a few days	remains infectious until 24h <u>after</u> begin of antibiotic treatment
ectious ononucleosis	4 ~ 6 weeks	- almost all adults are seropositive - 25% of adults are carriers - transmission via saliva (i.e. kissing)

21.7.) <u>IMMUNIZATIONS FOR INFANTS</u>

	birth	2m	4m	6m	15m	4~6y
hepatitis B	✓	✓		✓		
rotavirus		✓	✓	✓		
DTaP		✓	✓	✓	✓	✓
haemophilus influenzae pneumococcal		✓	✓	✓	✓	
iPV (Salk)		✓	✓		✓	✓
MMR + Varicella					✓	✓

Seasonal influenza vaccine is now recommended for all people !
(Minimum age 6 month).

Oral Polio (Sabin):
- live-attenuated
- lifelong immunity
- local gut and systemic immunity
- may cause paralytic disease

Injectable Polio (Salk):
- inactivated
- requires booster every 4-5 years
- minimal gut immunity
- no risk of paralytic disease

21.8.) RESPIRATORY TRACT INFECTIONS

croup	- usually viral - **gradual onset** - low fever - stridor improves with epinephrine	parainfluenza virus
epiglottitis	- **acute onset** - high fever - some relief with neck extension ("sniffing dog position") - "thumb-print sign" on x-ray	*hemophilus influenzae*
tracheitis	- **gradual onset** - high fever - subglottal narrowing	*Staph. aureus*
bronchiolitis	- children 2 to 6 months - variable fever - respiratory distress - rhonchi, wheezes, rales - does NOT respond to bronchodilators	**RSV (viral)**

21.9.) CROUP

Laryngotracheobronchitis - usually due to a virus

ASSESSMENT

- Hoarseness
- Barking cough
- Respiratory distress: *nasal flaring, grunting, intercostal retractions*
- Inspiratory stridor

IMPLEMENTATION

- Semi-Fowler's position
- Monitor respiratory status
- Cool fluids: fruit juice, soft drinks
- Have suction, intubation equipment and tracheostomy set on hand

MEDICATIONS:

- Decongestants, expectorants
- Antipyretics

21.10.) EPIGLOTTITIS

Inflammation of glottis – usually caused by bacterium *H. influenzae*

ASSESSMENT

- Fever
- Rapidly progressive respiratory distress
- Child appears "toxic"
- Characteristic posture: sitting upright, leaning forward, chin thrust out, mouth open, tongue protruding
- voice: muffled, thick
- croaking sound on inspiration

IMPLEMENTATION

- Medical emergency! Refer to physician immediately
- Otherwise same as for croup

MEDICATIONS:

- Antibiotics (bacterial cause!)

21.11.) <u>OTITIS MEDIA</u>

Middle ear infection – blocked eustachian tubes prevent drainage

---

ASSESSMENT
◊ Ear pain
◊ Impaired hearing
◊ Irritability
• Fever
• Otoscopy: bulging, opaque tympanic membrane

IMPLEMENTATION
• Apply local heat to promote drainage
• Watch for complications: - profound dizziness
                                   - meningitis

MEDICATIONS:
• Antibiotics
• Decongestants

MYRINGOTOMY:
• Incision of eardrum and insertion of small tube
• For severe, chronic cases

CLIENT EDUCATION
• Stress importance of <u>completing</u> antibiotic regimen, even if symptoms subside
• Use of vaporizers and decongestants during upper respiratory infections helps to prevent otitis media!

21.12.) <u>TONSILLITIS</u>

ASSESSMENT
- Soar throat
- Muffled voice
- Difficulty swallowing
- Enlarged cervical lymph nodes

IMPLEMENTATION
- Warm gargles

MEDICATION:
- Antibiotics if suspected streptococcal infection

POSTOPERATIVE:
- Soft diet, cool liquids for first 24h.
- Discourage coughing or blowing nose
- Position on side or stomach while sleeping to prevent aspiration
- Watch for signs of bleeding

<u>Feared complications of streptococcal infections:</u>

  ➢ *Rheumatic fever*
  ➢ *Glomerulonephritis*

21.13.) <u>REYE'S SYNDROME</u>

Acute fatty liver degeneration plus encephalopathy

➢ Very rare but severe complication of viral infections.
➢ More common if infection was treated with salicylates.

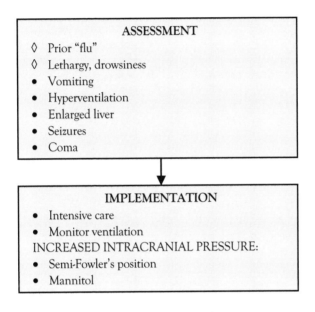

ASSESSMENT
◊ Prior "flu"
◊ Lethargy, drowsiness
• Vomiting
• Hyperventilation
• Enlarged liver
• Seizures
• Coma

IMPLEMENTATION
• Intensive care
• Monitor ventilation
INCREASED INTRACRANIAL PRESSURE:
• Semi-Fowler's position
• Mannitol

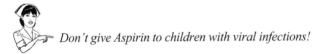

Don't give Aspirin to children with viral infections!

21.14.) RHEUMATIC FEVER

Complication of streptococcal infection → endocarditis → valve damage

major Jones criteria	• **carditis** • **polyarthritis** • **chorea** • **erythema marginatum** • **subcutaneous nodules**
minor Jones criteria	◊ arthralgia • fever • lab: elevated ESR

ASSESSMENT
◊ History of prior "strep throat"
• Jones criteria
• Throat culture to assess <u>present</u> infection with streptococci
• ASLO titer to confirm <u>past</u> infection with streptococci

↓

IMPLEMENTATION
• Alleviate joint pain
• Bed rest if fever or carditis are present
  (it may be necessary to maintain bed rest for several weeks)
• Auscultate heart sounds frequently
  (if extra sounds S3 or S4 develop → valve damage)
• Padded bed rails if chorea becomes severe
MEDICATIONS:
• Analgesics
• Steroids
• Antibiotics (check for history of penicillin allergy!)

↓

CLIENT EDUCATION
• Maintain good nutrition and hygiene
• Prophylactic penicillin before dental procedures or surgery
  • Seek immediate treatment of sore throat!

21.15.) JUVENILE RHEUMATOID ARTHRITIS

Chronic inflammatory disease – unknown cause

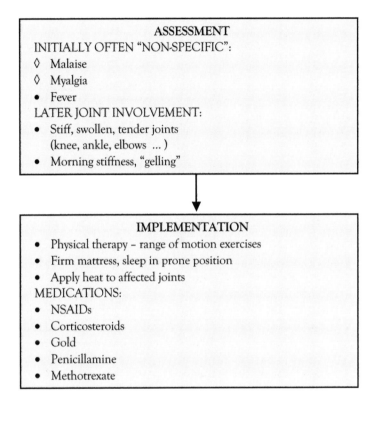

ASSESSMENT

INITIALLY OFTEN "NON-SPECIFIC":
◊ Malaise
◊ Myalgia
• Fever

LATER JOINT INVOLVEMENT:
• Stiff, swollen, tender joints
  (knee, ankle, elbows ...)
• Morning stiffness, "gelling"

IMPLEMENTATION

• Physical therapy – range of motion exercises
• Firm mattress, sleep in prone position
• Apply heat to affected joints

MEDICATIONS:
• NSAIDs
• Corticosteroids
• Gold
• Penicillamine
• Methotrexate

21.16.) CYSTIC FIBROSIS

Inability of exocrine glands to produce thin mucus - due to a simple gene defect.

Meconium ileus in newborns is often the earliest sign of cystic fibrosis.

ASSESSMENT
- Bulky, foul smelling stools (lack of pancreatic enzymes)
- Failure to thrive (due to malabsorption)
- Thick, tenacious mucus
- Frequent upper respiratory infections
- Sweat tastes salty

DIAGNOSTIC TEST:
- Sweat has abnormally high Cl⁻ concentration

↓

ANALYSIS
- Risk of infection
- Adequate bronchial clearance?
- Adequate nutrition?

↓

IMPLEMENTATION
- Chest percussion, postural drainage
- Breathing exercises
- Air humidifiers
- Encourage extra fluid intake
- Small, frequent, high-calorie meals

MEDICATIONS:
- Mucolytics
- Expectorants
- Replacement of digestive enzymes at meal-times

↓

CLIENT EDUCATION
Genetic counseling: <u>Autosomal recessive disease</u>:
→ 25% of offspring will have disease
→ 50% of offspring will be carriers of gene

21.17.) <u>LEUKEMIA</u>

Proliferation of immature white blood cells → depressed bone marrow function

---

ASSESSMENT

◊ Fatigue
◊ Anorexia
◊ Pale skin
- Anemia (low red blood cell production)
- Easy bruising (low platelet production)
- Susceptible to infections
  (immature white blood cells are ineffective)

IMPLEMENTATION

- Assist with diagnostic procedures:
  - CBC
  - bone marrow biopsy
  - lumbar puncture if signs of CNS involvement

CHEMOTHERAPY:
- Frequent rest periods
- Maintain protective isolation
- Monitor side effects of therapy
- Antiemetics for nausea

21.18.) <u>WILMS' TUMOR</u>

Malignant neoplasm of kidneys

ASSESSMENT

- Firm, painless abdominal mass
- Hematuria

IMPLEMENTATION

- Avoid palpation of abdomen after diagnosis is established

POSTOPERATIVE:
- Monitor side effects of chemotherapy

With resection and multi-agent chemotherapy: cure rates up to 90%

21.19.) <u>FEBRILE SEIZURES</u>

May occur with any cause of fever – about 3~5% of children affected

---

ASSESSMENT

- Fever, usually > 102°F
- Brief, generalized seizure

↓

IMPLEMENTATION

- Assess airways, breathing
- Antipyretics, cooling measures
- Protect from injury (padded side rails etc.)

Most infants have a single seizure episode only.
Risk of later epilepsy is 2~3%.

21.20.) <u>ENURESIS</u>

= bedwetting in children 5 years or older

ASSESSMENT

- Primary enuresis: never was able to control continence
- Secondary enuresis: happens after period of continence

↓

IMPLEMENTATION

- Avoid punishment, anger or blame
- Avoid creating feeling of guilt
- Positive reinforcement: rewards for dry nights
- No fluid intake 2-3h. before bed time
- Enuresis alarms are very effective
  (these are triggered by a few drops of urine)

21.21.) ADHD
= Attention Deficit Hyperactivity Disorder

➢ Major cause of learning disability
➢ More common in males

ASSESSMENT
- Easily distracted by external stimuli
- Shifts from one activity to another
- Difficulty remaining seated
- Difficulty listening
- Blurts out answers before questions are complete
- Difficulty awaiting his turn
- Often interrupts and intrudes on others
- Often engages in dangerous activities without considering possible consequences

---

IMPLEMENTATION
- Decrease external stimuli and distractions
- Provide stable, predictable environment
- Positive reinforcement of desired behavior

MEDICATIONS:
- Ritalin (=amphetamine-related psycho-stimulant)
  Probably grossly over-prescribed in US !!!

Children with ADHD have a paradoxical reaction to amphetamines: It calms them down!

PSYCHIATRY

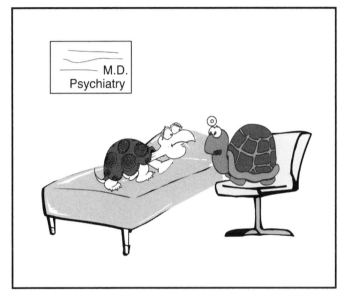

"Anytime a difficult situation arises, I suggest you simply
withdraw into your shell, rather than facing it."

22.1.) THE "DIFFICULT" CLIENT

CLIENT	YOUR BEST RESPONSE
withdrawn	- allow client to set pace - encourage social activities or games
depressed	- assess suicide potential - let client talk about personal problems - do not leave client alone
suicidal	**crisis intervention to asses suicide potential:** - ask for intent "Are you tired of living?..." - previous attempts? - specific plan? - social support system? - make a "No-Suicide Contract" !
anxious	- convey interest and care - don't "force" client - help client identify sources of anxiety - suggest relaxation techniques
violent	- remain calm and in control of the situation - give client space, avoid sudden movements - encourage verbal expression of anger - restrain or seclude if necessary

CLIENT	YOUR BEST RESPONSE
compulsive	- allow client to engage in rituals (these are used to cover up anxiety) - gradually limit length of time for rituals
manipulative	- set clear limits - hold client responsible for behavior
dependent	- don't reward dependent behavior - client should share responsibility for treatment
paranoid	- don't argue with client (simply state that you don't share his beliefs) - be reliable and consistent
delusional	- stay with client - don't argue about the reality of delusions - orient frequently to reality (place, situation) - assess potential for self-harm
somatization	- respect client and his problems (client is NOT faking!) - rule out physical basis for symptoms - help client express anxiety

22.2.) <u>DEFENSE MECHANISMS</u>

= unconscious mechanisms that serve to protect the ego

- ➢ **Conversion**
  A college student develops diarrhea on day of exam.

- ➢ **Regression**
  Returning to immature ways of dealing with stress: crying, tantrums...

- ➢ **Repression**
  Blocking of unacceptable urges and feelings from awareness.

- ➢ **Denial**
  Blocking of unacceptable information or perceptions from awareness.

- ➢ **Dissociation of affect**
  A girl laughs when telling about her failed exam.

- ➢ **Rationalization**
  Substituting an acceptable motive for attitudes or behavior for an unacceptable motive.

- ➢ **Reaction formation**
  You want to "kick your boss's ass" but end up kissing it.

- ➢ **Identification**
  A teenager dresses like Madonna and mimics her behavior.

- ➢ **Projection**
  "You are acting like a teenager, not I !"

- ➢ **Introjection**
  A boy yells at his dog like his father does to him.

- ➢ **Displacement**
  Client is upset about disease and yells at nurse. Nurse gets upset and yells at nursing assistant.

- ➢ **Undoing**
  "Magic": knocking on wood...

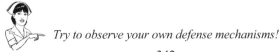

Try to observe your own defense mechanisms!

22.3.) SIGNS & SYMPTOMS

aphasia	- receptive[1] or expressive[2] language disorder
apraxia	- failure to do, despite intact motor function
agnosia	- failure to recognize
dementia	- gradual impairment of cognitive functions, memory - **Alzheimer dementia**: early memory loss - **multi-infarct dementia**: step-like decline
delirium	- **acute, organic, short lasting** - clouded consciousness - confusion, disorientation, anxiety - sometimes hallucinations
delusions	- persistent false belief despite invalidating evidence - grandeur - paranoia - somatic delusions
illusions	- misperception of external stimuli
hallucinations	- perception without external stimuli

[1] *Wernicke = difficulty to comprehend language*
[2] *Broca = difficulty to find the right word*

343

22.4.) MENTAL STATUS

appearance	- matches age? - grooming: appropriate? - posture: rigid? slumping? - skin: turgor? color? - sweating?
behavior	- eye contact? - agitated or relaxed? - cooperative or hostile? - withdrawn or dramatic? - speech: rapid or slow? slurred? - voice: loud or whisper?
affect and mood	- flat or intense? - appropriate to thought content?
thought process	- form: organized? circumstantial? incoherent? - content: obsessive? phobic? suicidal? **Neologisms:** invents new words [1] **Echolalia:** echoes words or sentences [1] **Word salad:** jumble of words without meaning [1] **Flight of ideas:** rapid switching from topic to topic [2] **Confabulation:** invents stories to fill memory gaps [3]
cognitive functions	- oriented to time? place? person? - memory (recent and remote)? - judgment and insight?

[1] *Schizophrenia*   [2] *Mania*   [3] *Korsakoff encephalopathy*

22.5.) <u>DELIRIUM</u> & <u>DEMENTIA</u>

delirium	◊ acute onset ◊ fluctuating consciousness ◊ disorientation ◊ optical hallucinations
dementia	◊ gradual onset ◊ no impairment of consciousness • loss of intellectual functions: memory, orientation, language

22.6.) <u>ALZHEIMER'S DISEASE</u>

Degeneration and atrophy of brain cortex → dementia

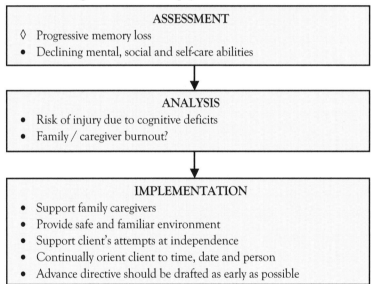

ASSESSMENT
◊ Progressive memory loss
• Declining mental, social and self-care abilities

ANALYSIS
• Risk of injury due to cognitive deficits
• Family / caregiver burnout?

IMPLEMENTATION
• Support family caregivers
• Provide safe and familiar environment
• Support client's attempts at independence
• Continually orient client to time, date and person
• Advance directive should be drafted as early as possible

Before making a diagnosis of Alzheimer's disease, treatable causes of dementia need to be ruled out such as: Parkinson's disease, hypo-thyroidism, and cerebrovascular diseases.

22.7.) DEMENTIA & DEPRESSION

Especially in the elderly depression and dementia may be difficult to distinguish. The following table should help:

	DEMENTIA	DEPRESSION
insight	*absent*	intact
recall of famous persons	*absent*	intact
vegetative signs	rare	*insomnia* *constipation* *anorexia*

22.8.) GRIEF & DEPRESSION

GRIEF	DEPRESSION
◊ initial: shock/denial ◊ illusions / hallucinations may occur	◊ feeling of hopelessness ◊ feeling of worthlessness
➤ low risk of suicide	➤ high risk of suicide

Abnormal grief:
- ◊ *continued thoughts about guilt and death*
- *marked psychomotor retardation*
- *marked functional impairment*

22.9.) PERSONALITY DISORDERS

1. Behavior is inflexible across a broad range of situations
2. Behavior is markedly deviant from cultural norms
3. Significant distress and impairment of functioning

dependent	◊ afraid of being helpless ◊ need to be cared for
compulsive	◊ fear of loss of control ◊ tries to control physician
passive-aggressive	◊ appears willing but is non-compliant
histrionic	◊ dramatic, emotional ◊ may display inappropriate sexual behavior
narcissistic	◊ feels better than others ◊ perfect self-image is threatened by disease
paranoid	◊ may blame nurse or others for disease
schizoid	◊ anxious, withdrawn (doesn't want close relationships)
borderline	◊ severe disorder! ◊ intense unstable relationships ◊ paranoia and suicidal behavior • features of psychoses

22.10.) ANXIETY DISORDERS

> Clients are distressed and know that their symptoms are irrational

phobia	◊ persistent excessive fear of specific objects or situations ◊ client knows that his fear is unrealistic
panic attack	◊ abrupt onset, peak within 10 min. ◊ palpitations, tachycardia ◊ sweating, trembling, shaking ◊ fear of dying • **derealization:** feeling of unreality of the external world • **depersonalization:** feeling of being detached from oneself
agoraphobia	◊ history of panic attacks ◊ patient avoids places were panic attack might occur (especially public places)
obsessive compulsive	• **obsessions:** recurrent thoughts • **compulsions:** repetitive behavior
posttraumatic stress disorder	◊ traumatic event in client's history ◊ may occur ANY time after event ◊ persists for > 1 month

22.11.) HYPOCHONDRIASIS & MALINGERING

hypochondriasis	◊ unrealistic interpretation of body signs
	◊ client believes to have serious disease that is unrecognized by family and physicians
factitious disorder	• intentional feigning of symptoms
	Motivation: - **to assume the "sick role"** [1]
malingering	• intentional feigning of symptoms
	Motivation: - **economic gain** - **avoiding legal responsibilities**

[1] _external_ incentives (such as economic gain or avoiding legal responsibilities) are absent!

Never _assume_ that a client with multiple symptoms must be hypochondriac or is malingering.

Always take the client's symptoms seriously !

22.12.) <u>MAJOR DEPRESSION</u>

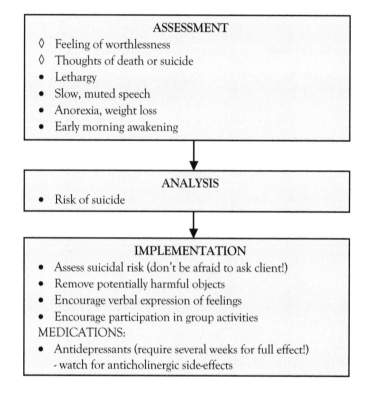

ASSESSMENT
◊ Feeling of worthlessness
◊ Thoughts of death or suicide
• Lethargy
• Slow, muted speech
• Anorexia, weight loss
• Early morning awakening

ANALYSIS
• Risk of suicide

IMPLEMENTATION
• Assess suicidal risk (don't be afraid to ask client!)
• Remove potentially harmful objects
• Encourage verbal expression of feelings
• Encourage participation in group activities
MEDICATIONS:
• Antidepressants (require several weeks for full effect!)
  - watch for anticholinergic side-effects

Anhedonia: *Inability to experience or express pleasure*
(normal state prior to taking NCLEX exam).

<u>ANTICHOLINERGIC SIDE-EFFECTS</u>:
◊ Blurred vision
◊ Dry mouth
◊ Constipation
• Urinary retention

22.13.) <u>BIPOLAR DISORDER</u>

➤ Manic episodes alternate with episodes of major depression
➤ Some clients have only manic episodes, no depressive episodes

---

ASSESSMENT
◊ Euphoria
◊ Grandiose ideas
• Uninhibited sexuality
• Buying sprees
• Psychomotor agitation

IMPLEMENTATION
• Low stimulus environment
• Provide frequent small meals, snacks
• Encourage physical activity as a means to "act out"
MEDICATIONS:
• Lithium
  - watch for signs of toxicity
  - monitor serum levels closely

<u>SIGNS OF LITHIUM TOXICITY</u>:
◊ Abdominal pain, nausea
• Hand tremor
• Ataxia, nystagmus
• Slurred speech

Lithium serum level should not exceed 1 mEq/L

22.14.) SCHIZOPHRENIA

ASSESSMENT

◊ Defect in reality testing
◊ Affect is incongruent (=does not match thoughts)
◊ Thoughts are tangential, circumstantial - loose associations
"POSITIVE SYMPTOMS":
◊ Delusions
◊ Hallucinations
"NEGATIVE SYMPTOMS":
◊ Flat affect
◊ Loss of interest
◊ Ambivalence
• Autism
CATATONIA:
• Waxy rigidity of muscles
• Client maintains bizarre postures

IMPLEMENTATION

• Establish trusting, honest relationship
• Maintain calm, consistent manner
• Don't challenge client's thought content
• Decrease environmental stimuli
MEDICATIONS:
• Neuroleptics
  - monitor for signs of tardive dyskinesia!

CLIENT EDUCATION

• Stress importance to comply with follow-up visits
• Encourage family support

TARDIVE DYSKINESIA:
(may occur after many months of treatment)
• Choreoathetosis
• Lateral movements of jaw
• Tongue protrusion

22.15.) DRUG ABUSE

Abuse:	- Recurrent use of drugs resulting in social failures (at home, school or work), legal problems or hazardous situations.
Dependence:	- Tolerance (needs larger and larger doses to achieve effect). - Withdrawal symptoms.

	INTOXICATION	WITHDRAWAL
alcohol	◊ euphoria ◊ disorientation • unsteady gait	◊ nausea ◊ delusions, hallucinations • delirium • tremor, seizures
barbiturates	◊ sedation	• delirium • epilepsy • coma, death
benzodiazepines	◊ antianxiety ◊ sedation	◊ anxiety ◊ irritability ◊ insomnia
amphetamines, cocaine	◊ arousal ◊ euphoria	◊ fatigue ◊ dysphoria
opioids	◊ euphoria ◊ apathy	• nausea, vomiting • sweating, fever • muscle aches
LSD	◊ hallucinations ◊ anxiety ◊ paranoid ideas	none

Blood alcohol: 1% → client is intoxicated
2% → client falls asleep, anesthesia
4% → inhibition of respiration, death

Legal limit: 0.08% for driving a car in USA.

353

22.16.) <u>EATING DISORDERS</u>

More common in females than in males

ANOREXIA NERVOSA	BULIMIA
◊ **refusal to maintain weight** (>15% below normal)	◊ lack of control over eating behavior ◊ **recurrent episodes of binge eating**
◊ intense fear of becoming fat ◊ disturbed body image	◊ persistent concern about body weight
• amenorrhea	• self-induced vomiting • abuse of laxatives, diuretics

---

IMPLEMENTATION
- Supportive and caring attitude
- Insist on adherence to therapeutic/nutritional plan (but allow client to feel being in control if possible)
- Provide high-calorie diet
- Monitor intake / output
- Weigh daily
- Watch for signs of non-compliance:
  - self-induced vomiting
  - hiding of food

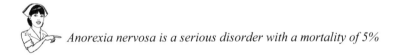

Anorexia nervosa is a serious disorder with a mortality of 5%

NURSING PHARMACOLOGY

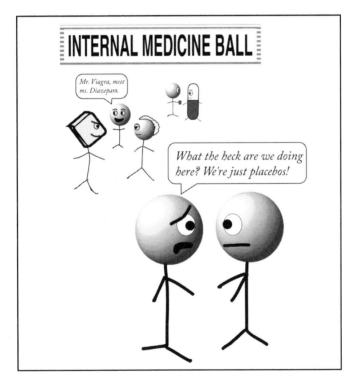

23.1.) SOME TRADEMARKS

The NCLEX requires you to know both generic drug names and trademarks. It is impossible to know them all! Here is a list of the 65 most commonly used and asked-for names. You can test whether you recognize the names by covering one half of these charts.

Keep practicing until they sound really familiar:

GENERIC NAME	TRADE NAME
NSAIDs	
- acetaminophen	- Tylenol
- ibuprofen	- Advil, Motrin
ANTIHYPERTENSIVES	
- propanolol	- Inderal
- nifedipine	- Procardia
- captopril	- Capoten
NITRATES	
- nitroglycerin	- Nitrostat
- ISDN	- Isordil
DIURETICS	
- furosemide	- Lasix
- thiazides	- Diuril, Esidrix
- spironolactone	- Aldactone
ANTIBIOTICS	
- penicillins	- PenVee, Amcill,…
- cephalosporins	- Keflex, Claforan,…
- sulfonamides	- Bactrim
- aminoglycosides	- Amikin, Streptomycin
- tetracycline	- Tetrex
- miconazole	- Monistat

GENERIC NAME	TRADE NAME
ANTI-LIPIDS	
- atorvastatin, simvastatin	- Lipitor, Zocor
- fenofibrate	- Tricor
HEART FAILURE	
- digoxin	- Lanoxin
- digitoxin	- Crystodigin
- dopamine	- Intropin
- dobutamine	- Dobutrex
ANTICOAGULANTS	
- heparin	- Heparin
- warfarin	- Coumadin
ANTIARRHYTHMICS	
- lidocaine	- Lidocaine, Xylocaine
- procainamide	- Pronestyl
- quinidine	- Cardioquin
DRUGS FOR ASTHMA	
- albuterol	- Proventil
- terbutaline	- Brethine
- theophylline	- Theo-Dur
DRUGS FOR PEPTIC ULCERS	
- antacids	- Maalox, Rolaids, Tums, …
- cimetidine	- Tagamet
- ranitidine	- Zantac
- omeprazole	- Prilosec
DRUGS USED IN OBSTETRICS	
- prostaglandins	- Prostin E2
- oxytocin	- Pitocin
- terbutaline	- Bricanyl

GENERIC NAME	TRADE NAME
ANXIOLYTICS - benzodiazepines - buspirone	- Valium, Librium, Ativan,… - BuSpar
ANTIDEPRESSANTS - tricyclics - SSRI [1]	- Elavil, Tofranil,… - Prozac, Zoloft,…
HYPNOTICS - barbiturates	- Nembutal, Seconal…
NEUROLEPTICS - fluphenazine - haloperidol - chlorpromazine - thioridazine	- Prolixin - Haldol - Thorazine - Mellaril
PARKINSON'S - levodopa + carbidopa - benztropine - biperiden	- Sinemet - Cogentin - Akineton
EPILEPSY - phenytoin	- Dilantin
CHEMOTHERAPY - doxorubicin - cyclophosphamide - vincristine - cisplatin	- Adriamycin - Cytoxan - Oncovin - Platinol

[1] *SSRI = selective serotonin reuptake inhibitors*

23.2.) SIDE-EFFECTS

"A drug without side-effects is a drug with no main effects."

The NCLEX exam tests your ability to practice safe nursing. It is important to be aware of side-effects of medications and to monitor for these in your clients. The charts in this section list the most important precautions and side-effects of common drugs that are tested on the NCLEX. For indications and usage of drugs see individual charts in the other chapters ("Implementation").

FAMOUS SIDE EFFECT:	CAUSED BY:
anaphylactic shock	- penicillin - foreign proteins
hepatotoxicity	- isoniazid - halothane
renal toxicity	- phenacetin - other NSAIDs - cyclosporin
ototoxicity	- aminoglycosides
drug-induced lupus	- procainamide - hydralazine
photosensitivity (skin)	- tetracyclines - sulfonamides - sulfonylureas
bone marrow suppression	- chloramphenicol - ganciclovir - zidovudine (AZT)

23.3.) ANTIBIOTICS

➢ All antibiotics may cause diarrhea due to disruption of normal flora.

	MAJOR SIDE EFFECTS	NURSING INTERVENTIONS
penicillins	allergic reactions: - maculopapular rash - anaphylactic shock	- watch for rash, fever and chills - be prepared to treat anaphylaxis
cephalosporins	allergic reactions	- check patient history: avoid in patients with known penicillin allergy (cross reactivity)
sulfonamides	renal toxicity	- best absorbed on empty stomach - increase fluid intake
aminoglycosides	renal toxicity ototoxicity	- increase fluid intake - watch for tinnitus, vertigo or hearing loss
tetracyclines	bind with calcium	- give at least <u>2</u> hours before or after ingesting milk - don't give in 2nd half of pregnancy or to children < 8 years (risk of tooth discoloration)
isoniazid (antitubercular)	hepatotoxicity peripheral neuropathy	- watch for loss of appetite, jaundice, dark urine - monitor liver function tests - avoid alcohol
rifampin (antitubercular)	hepatotoxicity orange color urine	- teach client that orange coloration is normal effect
ethambutol	impaired vision	- evaluate client's vision and color discrimination

360

➤ NSAIDs inhibit prostaglandin synthesis and may cause acute erosive gastritis and bleeding. Discourage "routine" use.

	MAJOR SIDE EFFECTS	NURSING INTERVENTIONS
aspirin	GI distress, occult bleeding suppresses platelet function may cause Reye's syndrome	- give with meals or milk - don't give within 1 week of surgery (risk of bleeding) - don't give to children with viral infections
acetaminophen	liver toxicity with overdose	- monitor liver enzymes for 1 week in case of overdose
ibuprofen	GI distress	- give with meals or milk
phenylbutazone	bone marrow suppression, anemia	- monitor CBC - should not be used for more than 1 week
indomethacin	CNS: dizziness, lightheadedness blurred vision	- regular eye exam if used for long-term therapy

SIGNS OF SALICYLATE INTOXICATION:
- **Mild:** tinnitus, central hyperventilation
- **Severe:** respiratory plus metabolic acidosis

REYE'S SYNDROME:
- Avoid aspirin in children with viral infections → risk of fulminant hepatitis & cerebral edema

23.5.) CORTICOSTEROIDS

	MAJOR SIDE EFFECTS	NURSING INTERVENTIONS
cortisone, dexamethasone	Cushing's syndrome adrenal suppression skin atrophy	CREAMS: - don't apply to broken skin - don't apply near eyes SYSTEMIC: - monitor for edema, signs of infection - avoid immobility (increased risk of osteoporosis) - never discontinue abruptly

23.6.) ANTIHYPERTENSIVE DRUGS

	CONTRAINDICATIONS	NURSING INTERVENTIONS
propanolol (β-blockers)	diabetes asthma peripheral vascular disease	- watch client: dizziness and fatigue increase risk of injury - advise client NOT to discontinue abruptly (risk of rebound hypertension, angina and MI)
nifedipine (Ca²⁺ antagonists)	congestive heart failure	- advise client NOT to discontinue abruptly (risk of rebound hypertension, angina and MI)
captopril (ACE inhibitors)	pregnancy	- advise client to stand up slowly (orthostatic hypotension is a common problem)

	MAJOR SIDE EFFECTS	NURSING INTERVENTIONS
nitroglycerin, ISDN	headache, dizziness orthostatic hypotension	- occasional headache: aspirin or acetaminophen - frequent headache: may have to adjust dosage - instruct client to rise slowly from sitting position - instruct client to protect drug from light, heat and moisture

23.8.) DIURETICS

	MAJOR SIDE EFFECTS	NURSING INTERVENTIONS
furosemide **(loop diuretics)**	hypokalemia	- recommend foods rich in potassium: bananas, prunes… - watch for signs of hypokalemia: muscle weakness, cramps
thiazides	hypokalemia hyperglycemia	- recommend foods rich in potassium: bananas, prunes… - watch for signs of hypokalemia: muscle weakness, cramps - monitor blood glucose
spironolactone **(potassium sparing)**	gynecomastia menstrual irregularity	- client needs to be advised of possible endocrine effects - teach client to avoid excessive dietary potassium
mannitol **(osmotic diuretic)**	transient plasma volume increase	- monitor vital signs and central venous pressure

 Hypokalemia potentiates digitalis toxicity !

363

23.9.) CONGESTIVE HEART FAILURE

Ⓐ Inotropic drugs: increased strength of cardiac contractions → increased stroke volume → increased cardiac output

	MAJOR SIDE EFFECTS	NURSING INTERVENTIONS
digoxin, digitoxin	low therapeutic index !!! (=high risk of toxicity)	- take apical pulse for full minute, monitor ECG - do not give if heart rate is low! - **monitor potassium levels** (risk of enhanced toxicity!)
dobutamine, dopamine	hypertension, headache, angina	- alert physician if arrhythmia, chest pain or dyspnea occur

DIGITALIS TOXICITY:

extracardiac: - nausea, abdominal pain
- fatigue
- confusion, disorientation
- color misperception: yellow halos

cardiac: - AV block, arrhythmias

Toxicity of DIGITALIS is enhanced by:
- Hypokalemia
- Alkalosis

23.10.) ANTICOAGULANTS

	ANTAGONIST (IN CASE OF OVERDOSE)	NURSING INTERVENTIONS
heparin (immediate effect)	protamine sulfate	- do not give IM (→ hematoma and pain) - watch for bleeding, bruises - teach client not to take aspirin - monitor partial thromboplastin time (PTT)
warfarin (4–5 days for full effect)	vitamin K	- watch for bleeding, bruises - teach client not to take aspirin - if ongoing therapy: client should carry medical alert card - monitor prothrombin time (PT) Drugs that enhance action: - antibiotics, salicylates, tolbutamide Drugs that reduce action: - barbiturates, oral contraceptives
streptokinase, urokinase (to dissolve thrombi)	aminocaproic acid	- risk of severe bleeding: have blood available for transfusion

23.11.) ANTIARRHYTHMIC DRUGS

⊁ All antiarrhythmics have the potential to worsen arrhythmia → bradycardias, tachycardias, hypotension!
⊁ Instruct client to take exactly as prescribed

	MAJOR SIDE EFFECTS	NURSING INTERVENTIONS
procainamide	reversible lupus erythematosus	- discontinue under medical supervision if lupus occurs
phenytoin [1]	gingiva hyperplasia	- teach proper mouth and dental care
quinidine	potentiates digitoxin toxicity	- monitor apical heart rate and blood pressure - monitor ECG

[1] *also used as anticonvulsant*

	MAJOR SIDE EFFECTS	NURSING INTERVENTIONS
albuterol, terbutaline (β2-agonists)	tremor dizziness palpitations	- do not exceed prescribed dose - notify physician if client becomes non-responsive to usual dose
theophylline	arrhythmias, seizures	- monitor vital signs - maintenance: teach client to take at regular intervals during day
corticosteroids	Cushing's syndrome	- do not discontinue abruptly (may trigger adrenal insufficiency crisis!)

23.13.) PEPTIC ULCERS

	MAJOR SIDE EFFECTS	NURSING INTERVENTIONS
antacids (for symptomatic relief)	Al-containing: constipation Mg-containing: diarrhea	- take after meals, at bed-time or whenever needed
cimetidine (H₂ blockers)	anti-androgenic	- don't use for minor digestive complaints
omeprazole (proton pump inhibitor)	rare side effects	- give in morning before breakfast

23.14.) SEX-HORMONES

➢ Oral contraceptives are no substitute for safe sex practices!

	SIDE EFFECTS	NURSING INTERVENTIONS
estrogens	- nausea - vomiting - breast tenderness - skin pigmentation - hypertension - breakthrough bleeding	- discourage smoking! - discontinue immediately if pregnancy suspected - may need to adjust dosage of other common medications (oral anticoagulants, diazepam, barbiturates, others...)
progesterones	- weight gain - depression - hirsutism	- discontinue immediately if pregnancy suspected

Risks of Oral Contraceptives:

- Thrombosis, embolism (especially in smokers!)
- Benign adenoma of the liver
- Vaginal cancer in daughters of mothers who received DES

- May slightly increase risk of breast cancer
- Decreases risk of endometrial cancer

23.15.) DRUGS USED IN OBSTETRICS

	MAJOR SIDE EFFECTS	NURSING INTERVENTIONS
PGE$_2$ (for cervical ripening)	uterine hyperstimulation, pain	
oxytocin (stimulates uterus)	hypertension, arrhythmia fetal bradycardia	- monitor vital signs closely - discontinue if signs of fetal distress
terbutaline (relaxes uterus)	tachycardia dyspnea, chest pain	- monitor ECG and vital signs
magnesium sulfate (prevents seizures)	hypotension, bradycardia respiratory depression muscle hyporeflexia	- monitor vital signs closely - monitor knee jerk reflex - keep calcium gluconate at hand as antidote

23.16.) ANXIOLYTIC DRUGS

➢ Anxiolytic drugs should be used short-term only.
➢ Abrupt withdrawal may cause delirium and seizures!

	MAJOR SIDE EFFECTS	NURSING INTERVENTIONS
benzodiazepines	drowsiness, sedation	- don't drive car - avoid alcohol - discontinue by slowly tapering off
buspirone	hypotension, tachycardia tremors	- monitor blood pressure, pulse

23.17.) HYPNOTIC DRUGS

	MAJOR SIDE EFFECTS	NURSING INTERVENTIONS
barbiturates	tolerance and physical dependence	- use only for few days at the most - don't drive car - discontinue by slowly tapering off
chloral hydrate	epigastric pain REM rebound	- don't drive car - discontinue by slowly tapering off

23.18.) ANTIDEPRESSANTS

⋏ Suicide assessment (ask client directly). Suicide risk often increases initially during treatment!
⋏ Antidepressants usually require 3 to 4 weeks for full therapeutic effect.

	MAJOR SIDE EFFECTS	NURSING INTERVENTIONS
tricyclics: amitriptyline amoxapine desipramine etc.	agranulocytosis orthostatic hypotension **anticholinergic side effects:** blurred vision, dry mouth constipation urinary retention	- monitor CBC - advise client to stand up slowly - increase fluid and fiber intake
fluoxetine (Prozac)	fewer anticholinergic effects	- increase fluid intake
MAO inhibitors	risk of hypertensive crisis	- avoid foods with high tyramine content: (cheese, yogurt, beer, red wine)

23.19.) LITHIUM

➢ Lithium has an extremely low therapeutic index and needs to be monitored closely.

	SIGNS & SYMPTOMS	NURSING INTERVENTIONS
"normal" side-effects	- mild nausea - thirst	- teach client that nausea and thirst will subside after a few days - avoid low-sodium diet - instruct client to carry identification card (side effects may be mistaken for alcohol intoxication) - do not discontinue drug abruptly
early intoxication 1.5 - 2 mEq/L	- abdominal pain, vomiting - hand tremor - ataxia, nystagmus - slurred speech	- monitor serum level
severe intoxication > 2 mEq/L	- persistent vomiting - blurred vision - hyperactive tendon reflexes - convulsions, coma, death	- treat as medical emergency

Low-salt diet decreases lithium excretion → enhanced toxicity

	MAJOR SIDE EFFECTS	NURSING INTERVENTIONS
chlorpromazine, fluphenazine (phenothiazines)	- more anticholinergic side effects - fewer extrapyramidal side effects	- monitor for dyskinesia
haloperidol (butyrophenones)	- more extrapyramidal side effects - fewer anticholinergic side effects	- monitor for dyskinesia
clozapine	- bone marrow suppression - fewer extrapyramidal side effects	- monitor for dyskinesia - monitor CBC

DYSKINESIAS CAUSED BY NEUROLEPTICS

Acute dystonia occurs within hours of administration:
- stiff neck, jaw dislocation, tongue protrusion
- usually disappears (tolerance)

Parkinsonism occurs within weeks to months of treatment:
- muscle stiffness, cogwheel rigidity, shuffling, drooling
- usually disappears (tolerance)

Tardive dyskinesia occurs after many months of treatment:
- jerky movements, tongue protrusion, lateral movements of jaw
- fine, worm-like tongue movements are an early sign
- may be irreversible!

23.21.) PARKINSON'S DISEASE

	MAJOR SIDE EFFECTS	NURSING INTERVENTIONS
levodopa + carbidopa (dopaminergic)	nausea, vomiting dyskinesia depression, mood changes	- take with food to decrease GI irritation - urine darkening is quite harmless
benztropine, biperiden (anticholinergic)	dry mouth mydriasis tachycardia constipation urinary retention	- increase fluid and fiber intake to avoid constipation

"On-off" phenomenon: Sudden recurrence of Parkinsonian symptoms.

23.22.) CHEMOTHERAPY

⋏ All anticancer drugs cause nausea, vomiting, hair loss and bone marrow suppression (→ high risk of infections)

	MAJOR SIDE EFFECTS	NURSING INTERVENTIONS
doxorubicin	cardiotoxic	- monitor vital signs and heart rate for arrhythmia
cyclophosphamide	hemorrhagic cystitis	- encourage fluid intake - report any unexpected bleeding , hematuria or dysuria
cisplatin	renal toxicity	- encourage fluid intake
vincristine	peripheral neuropathy	- tell client to report numbness or tingling in finger or toes
L-asparaginase	allergic reactions	- skin test to assess allergic reaction before first use - watch for signs of anaphylactic shock when administering

375

CONVERSIONS

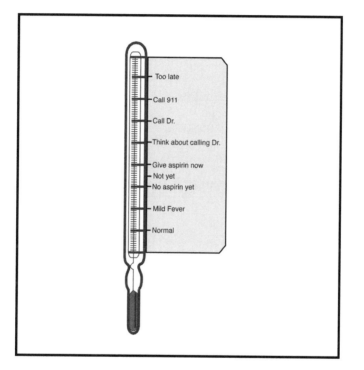

Thermometer Made Ridiculously Simple

24.1.) METRIC SYSTEM

1 kg	1,000 g
1 g	1,000 mg
1 L	10 dL 1,000 mL
1 dL	100 mL
1 mL	1 cc

24.2.) APOTHECARY SYSTEM

1 grain	65 mg
1 dram	60 grains = 3.9 g
1 ounce	8 drams = 31.1 g
15 drops	1 mL
1 fluid dram	60 drops = 4 mL
1 fluid ounce	8 fluid drams = 32 mL

24.3.) <u>HOUSEHOLD SYSTEM</u>

1 teaspoon		~5 mL
1 tablespoon	½ ounce	~15 mL
1 cup	8 ounces	~240 mL
1 pint	16 ounces	473 mL
1 quart	2 pints	946 mL
1 gallon	4 quarts	3,785 mL

 US fluid ounce = 29.6 mL

24.4.) <u>TEMPERATURE CONVERSION</u>

CELSIUS	FAHRENHEIT
37.0	98.6
37.5	99.5
38.0	100.4
38.5	101.3
39.0	102.2
39.5	103.1
40.0	104.0

°F → °C: Subtract 32, then divide by 1.8
°C → °F: Multiply by 1.8, then add 32

NORMAL RANGE:

oral	36.4 ~ 37.4 °C	97.6 ~ 99.3 °F
rectal	36.2 ~ 37.8 °C	97.0 ~ 100.0 °F
axillary	35.9 ~ 36.7 °C	96.6 ~ 98.0 °F

24.5.) PRESCRIPTIONS

ad lib.	as desired
p.r.n.	if required
stat	immediately
c̲ (cum)	with
s̲ (sine)	without
b.i.d.	two times daily
t.i.d.	three times a day
q.i.d.	four times a day
q.h.	every hour
q.d.	every day
q.o.d.	every other day
a.c.	before meals
p.c.	after meals
s̲s̲	one-half

ABBREVIATIONS

a/w	associated with	GI	gastrointestinal
ABG	arterial blood gases	HLA	human leukocyte antigens
ACE	angiotensin converting enzyme	ICP	intracranial pressure
ACTH	adrenocorticotropic hormone	IDDM	insulin-dependent diabetes mellitus
ADH	antidiuretic hormone	IF	intrinsic factor
ALL	acute lymphoblastic leukemia	INR	international normalized ratio
ALT	alanine aminotransferase	ISDN	isosorbide dinitrate
AML	acute myeloblastic leukemia	ITP	idiopathic thrombocytopenic purpura
ASLO	antistreptolysin-O	IVP	intravenous pyelogram
AST	aspartate aminotransferase	LDH	lactate dehydrogenase
BMI	body mass index	LH	luteinizing hormone
BP	blood pressure	MAO	monoamine oxidase
BUN	blood urea nitrogen	MCP	metacarpophalangeal joint
CBC	complete blood count	MI	myocardial infarction
CEA	carcinoembryonic antigen	NIDDM	noninsulin-dependent diabetes mellitus
CHD	coronary heart disease	NPO	nothing per os
CLL	chronic lymphocytic leukemia	NSAID	nonsteroidal anti-inflammatory drugs
CML	chronic myelocytic leukemia	PACU	post-anesthesia care unit
COPD	chronic obstructive pulmonary disease	PEEP	positive end-expiratory pressure
CPK	creatine phosphokinase	PIP	proximal interphalangeal joint
CSF	cerebrospinal fluid	PSA	prostate specific antigen
CVP	central venous pressure	PT	prothrombin time
DES	diethylstilbestrol	PTH	parathormone
DHT	dihydrotestosterone	PTT	partial thromboplastin time
DIC	disseminated intravascular coagulation	RBC	red blood cells
DIP	distal interphalangeal joint	REM	rapid eye movements
DTaP	diphtheria, tetanus, acellular Pertussis	RSV	respiratory syncytial virus
DVT	deep venous thrombosis	STD	sexually transmitted disease
ELISA	enzyme linked immunosorbent assay	TBC	tuberculosis
ERCP	endoscopic retrograde cholangio-pancreatography	TIA	transient ischemic attack
		TSH	thyroid stimulating hormone
ESR	erythrocyte sedimentation rate	TTP	thrombotic thrombocytopenic purpura
FSH	follicle stimulating hormone	VDRL	Venereal Disease Research Laboratory
GH	growth hormone	WBC	white blood cells

INDEX

ABC of trauma, **16.1**
Abdominal pain, **6.4, 6.21**
Abdominal trauma, **16.5**
Abortion, **18.16**
Abruptio placentae, 18.4, 18.13, **18.19**
ACE inhibitors, 23.6
Acetaminophen, 6.13, 23.4
Acid/base, **3.2**
Acidosis, 3.2
Acidosis, metabolic, **3.5**
Acidosis, respiratory, **3.4**
Acne, **15.3**
Acromegaly, **11.4**
ACTH, 11.2, 11.3, 5.15
Actinic keratosis,15.8
Addison's disease, 3.11, **11.7**
Addisonian crisis, **11.8**
ADH, 5.15, 11.1
ADHD, **21.21**
Adriamycin, 23.1
Advil, 23.1
Aflatoxin, 6.13
Agnosia, 22.3
Agoraphobia, 22.10
AIDS, **8.2, 8.3**
Airway clearance, 1.4
Akineton, 23.1
Albumin, 10.1
Albuterol, 23.12
Alcohol, 6.13, 20.11, 22.15
Aldactone, 23.1
Aldosterone, 11.1
Alkalosis, 3.2
Alkalosis, metabolic, **3.7**
Alkalosis, respiratory, **3.6**
ALL, 10.7
Altitude sickness, **16.14**
Alzheimer's disease, **22.6**
Amcill, 23.1
Amenorrhea, **17.5, 17.6**

Amikin, 23.1
Aminocaproic acid, 23.10
Aminoglycosides, 23.3
Amitriptyline, 23.18
AML, 10.7
Amniocentesis, 18.7
Amnion band syndrome, 20.1
Amoxapine, 23.18
Amphetamines, 22.15
Amputation, **12.12**
Amyotrophic lateral sclerosis, **13.15**
Anemia, **10.4**
Anencephaly, 20.12
Aneurysms, **4.26**
Angina pectoris, **4.5, 4.7**
Animal bites, 16.15
Ankylosing spondylitis, 12.6
Anorexia nervosa, 6.1, 22.16
Antacids, 23.13
Antiarrhythmic drugs, **23.11**
Antibiotics, **23.3**
Antibodies, 9.3
Anticholinergic side-effects, 22.12
Anticoagulants, **23.10**
Antidepressants, **23.18**
Antihypertensive drugs, **23.6**
Anxiety, 1.4, 22.1, **22.10**
Anxiolytic drugs, **23.16**
Aortic dissection, 16.4
Aortic regurgitation, 4.20
Aortic stenosis, 4.20
Apgar score, **20.2**
Aphasia, 22.3
Apothecary system, **24.2**
Appendicitis, 6.21, **6.22**
Apraxia, 22.3
ARDS, **5.14**
Arrhythmia, **4.10**
Arterial blood gases, 3.2

Arterial embolism, 4.23
Arteriosclerosis, 4.23, **4.24**
Arthritis, **12.2**
Asbestosis, 5.13
Aspirin, 23.4
Asterixis, 6.10, 13.1
Asthma, 5.9, **5.12, 23.12**
Ataxia, 13.1
Athetosis, 13.1
Ativan, 23.1
Atrial flutter, 4.10
Autonomic nervous system, **13.4**
AV block, 4.10
AV node, 4.1
AZT, 8.3

B12 deficiency, 10.4
Babinski reflex, 20.4
Bactrim, 23.1
Barbiturates, 22.15, 23.17
Barrel chest, 5.2
Basal ganglia, 13.3
Basilar skull fractures, 16.3
Bell's palsy, **13.16**
Benzodiazepines, 22.15, 23.16
Benztropine, 23.21
Beta-agonists, 23.12
Beta-blockers, 23.6
Biliary colic, 6.16
Bilirubin, 6.11
Biot respiration, 5.2
Biperiden, 23.21
Bipolar disorder, **22.13**
Birth defects, **20.12**
Birth trauma, **20.1**
Bladder rupture, 16.6
Bleeding disorders, **10.11**
Blindness, **14.3**
Blood, **10.1**
Blood cells, **10.2**
Blood pressure, 1.10, 4.1
Blood products, **10.5**
Blood vessels, **4.23**, 13.4
Bloody show, 18.13
Body mass index, 6.1
Bone marrow suppression, 23.2

Borderline personality, 22.9
Brain stem, 13.3
Breast abscess, 17.11
Breast cancer, 17.11, 17.12, **17.13**
Breast-feeding, 18.23
Breast milk, 19.1
Breast self-exam, **17.14**
Breath odors, 5.2
Breathing pattern, 1.4, **5.2**
Breech presentation, 18.9
Brethine, 23.1
Bricanyl, 23.1
Broca, 22.3
Bronchiolitis, 21.8
Bronchopneumonia, 5.7
Brudzinski's sign, 9.2
Buck's traction, 16.11
Buffalo hump, 11.5
Bulimia, 22.16
BUN, 7.5
Burns, **16.12**
BuSpar, 23.1
Buspirone, 23.16
Butyrophenones, 23.20

Calcium antagonists, 23.6
Calcium levels, **3.14**
Cancer, **1.9**
Cancer screening, **1.8**
Candida albicans, 6.2
Canes, **12.13**
Capoten, 23.1
Captopril, 23.6
Caput succedaneum, 20.1
Carbon tetrachloride, 6.13
Cardiac output, 1.4, 4.1
Cardiomyopathy, **4.21**
Cardioquin, 23.1
Carpal tunnel syndrome, **12.10**
Casts, **16.10**
Cataract, **14.2**
Central nervous system, **13.3**
Cephalhematoma, 20.1
Cephalosporins, 23.3
Cerebellum, 13.3
Cerebral palsy, **20.14**

Cervical cancer, **17.15**
Cervical mucus, 17.1
Cesarean section, **18.18**
Cesium sticks, 1.9
Chadwick's sign, 18.2
Chalazion, 14.5
Chancroid, 8.1
Charcot's triad, 6.16
Cheilosis, 2.11, 6.2
Chemotherapy, 1.9, **23.22**
Chest pain, **4.5, 4.6**
Chest trauma, **16.4**
Chest tubes, 5.5
Cheyne stokes respiration, 5.2
Chickenpox, 21.5, 21.6
Child abuse, **19.6**
Chlamydia, 8.1
Chloasma, 18.2
Chloral hydrate, 23.17
Chlorpromazine, 6.13, 23.20
Cholangitis, 6.16
Cholecystitis, 6.4, 6.16, **6.17**
Cholelithiasis, 6.16
Cholestasis, 6.12
Cholesterol, 2.4, 4.4
Chorea, 13.1
Chronic bronchitis, 5.9, **5.10**
Chvostek sign, 3.16
Cimetidine, 23.13
Cisplatin, 23.22
Claforan, 23.1
Cleft lip, 20.12
Client's needs, **1.5**
CLL, 10.8
Clozapine, 23.20
CML, 10.8
Coagulation defects, 10.11
Cocaine, 22.15
Cogentin, 23.1
Cognitive functions, 22.4
Cogwheel rigidity, 13.1
Colle's fracture, 16.7
Colorectal cancer, **6.28**
Coma, 13.2
Common cold, 5.6
Communication skills, **1.1**

Compartment syndrome, 16.7
Compulsion, 22.1
Concussion, 16.3
Condoms, 17.2
Confabulation, 22.4
Conization, 17.15
Conjunctivitis, **14.4**
Conn syndrome, 3.11, **11.6**
Constipation, 1.4
Contraception, **17.2**
Contusion, 16.3
Conversion, 22.2
Coombs' test, 10.3
COPD, **5.9**
Coping, ineffective, 1.4
Cord prolapse, **18.20**
Coronary arteries, 4.5
Coronary heart disease, **4.4**
Corticosteroids, 11.1, **23.5**
Coumadin, 23.1
Crackles, 5.3
Cranial nerves, **13.5**
Creatinine, 7.5
Crohn's disease, **6.25**
Croup, 21.8, **21.9**
Crutches, **12.13**
Cryoprecipitate, 10.5
Cryptorchidism, **21.4**
Crystodigin, 23.1
Cushing's disease, **11.5**
Cyclophosphamide, 23.22
Cystic fibrosis, **21.16**
Cystitis, 7.3
Cytoxan, 23.1

Decerebrate posture, 13.1
Decorticate posture, 13.1
Defense mechanisms, **22.2**
Dehydration, **3.9**
Delirium, 22.3, **22.5**
Delusions, 22.1, 22.3
Dementia, 22.3, **22.5, 22.7**
DeMusset sign, 4.20
Denial, 22.2
Dependent personality, 22.9
Depersonalization, 22.10

Depression, 22.1, **22.7**, **22.8**, **22.12**
Derealization, 22.10
Dermatitis, **15.2**
Desipramine, 23.18
Dexamethasone, 23.5
Diabetes mellitus, **11.11**
Diabetic diet, 2.6
Diabetic mothers, infants of, 20.5
Diaper dermatitis, **21.3**
Diarrhea, 1.4, **6.20**
DIC, **10.14**
Diet, **2.1**, 2.2, 2.3, 2.4, 2.5, 2.6, 2.7, 2.8, 2.9
Diffusion, **3.1**
Digital rectal exam, 1.8
Digitalis, 23.9
Digitalis toxicity, 4.12, 23.9
Dilantin, 23.1
Diphenylhydantoin, 20.11
Displacement, 22.2
Disseminated intravascular coagulation, **10.14**
Dissociation, 22.2
Diuretics, **23.8**
Diuril, 23.1
Diverticulitis, 6.21, **6.23**
Dobutamine, 23.9
Dobutrex, 23.1
Dopamine, 23.9
Dosage calculation, **2.12**
Down's syndrome, **20.15**
Doxorubicin, 23.22
Dram, 24.2
Dressing, 1.13
Drowning, **16.13**
Drug abuse, **22.15**
Drugs, in pregnancy, 20.11
DUB, 17.4
Duchenne's muscle atrophy, 13.1
Duodenal ulcer, 6.4, 6.9
Dysfunctional uterine bleeding, 17.4
Dyskinesias, 23.20
Dysmenorrhea, **17.7**

Ears, **14.8**
Eating disorders, **22.16**

Ecchymoses, 6.10
ECG, 4.2
Echolalia, 22.4
Ejaculation, 13.4
Elavil, 23.1
Emphysema, 5.9, **5.11**
Endocarditis, **4.22**
Endometrial cancer, **17.17**
Endometriosis, **17.8**
Enuresis, **21.20**
Epidural hematoma, 16.3
Epiglottitis, 21.8, **21.10**
Epilepsy, **13.17**, 21.19
Erb-Duchenne paralysis, 20.1
Erection, 13.4
Erikson, 19.3
Erythema infectiosum, 21.5
Erythrocytes, **10.3**
Erythrocytosis, 10.2
Erythropoietin, 7.1
Esidrix, 23.1
Esophageal atresia, **20.16**
Esophageal varices, **6.7**
Esophagitis, 6.4, **6.5**
Estrogen replacement therapy, 17.10
Estrogen, 6.13, 11.1, 23.14
Ethambutol, 23.3
Exercise, 2.1
Eyes, **14.1**

Factitious disorder, 22.11
Failure to thrive, **19.5**
Fallot's tetralogy, 20.13
False labor, 18.12
Farmer's lung, 5.13
Farsightedness, 14.1
Fear, 1.4
Febrile seizures, **21.19**
Ferning, 17.1
Fetor hepaticus, 6.10
Fetus, **18.9**, **18.10**
Fetus, heart rate, **18.11**
Fetus, stage of, 18.14
Fibrocystic change, **17.12**
Flail chest, 16.4
Flight of ideas, 22.4

Fluid volume deficit, 1.4
Fluoxetine, 23.18
Fluphenazine, 23.20
Folate deficiency, 10.4
Fowler's position, 1.7
Fractures, **16.7**
Fresh frozen plasma, 10.5
Freud, 19.3
FSH, 5.15, 11.2
Furosemide, 23.8

Gallbladder, **6.16**
Gallon, 24.3
Gas exchange, 1.4
Gastric ulcer, 6.4, 6.9
Gastritis, **6.8**
Gastrointestinal bleeding, **6.3**
Genital herpes, 8.1
Genital warts, 8.1
Genitourinary trauma, **16.6**
German measles, 21.5, 21.6
Giant cell arteritis, 4.27
Glasgow coma scale, **13.2**
Glaucoma, **14.6**
Glomeruli, 7.1
Glomerulonephritis, **7.6**
Glossitis, 6.2
Gonadotrope hormones, 11.1
Gonorrhea, 8.1
Gout, **12.5**
Gower's sign, 13.1
Grain, 24.2
Graves' disease, 11.9
Grief, 1.4, **22.8**
Growth hormone, 11.3
Guillain-Barré syndrome, 13.12
Gynecomastia, 6.10

H₂ blockers, 23.13
Haldol, 23.1
Hallucinations, 22.3
Haloperidol, 23.20
Hand washing, 1.6
HBe-Ag, 6.11
HBs-Ag, 6.11
HDL, 4.4

Head trauma, **16.3**
Headache, **13.7**
Health promotion, **2.1**
Hearing loss, 14.8
Heart defects, **20.13**
Heart failure, **4.12, 4.13, 23.9**
Heart valves, **4.20**
Heberden's nodes, 12.1
Hegar's sign, 18.2
Helicobacter pylori, 6.9
Hematemesis, 6.3, 6.7
Hematochezia, 6.3
Hematocrit, 10.3
Hemianopia, 11.4
Hemodialysis, 7.8
Hemoglobin, 10.3
Hemolysis, 10.4
Hemophilia, **10.13**
Hemorrhoids, **6.24**
Hemothorax, 16.4
Hemotympanum, 16.3
Henoch Schönlein, 4.27
Heparin, 23.1, 23.10
Hepatic encephalopathy, 6.10
Hepatitis, **6.15**
Hepatotoxicity, 23.2
Herniated disk, **12.9**
Herpes zoster, 21.5
Hiatal hernia, **6.6**
Hip dysplasia, **20.20**
Hirschsprung's disease, **20.19**
Histrionic personality, 22.9
Hodgkin's disease, 10.10
Household system, **24.3**
Huntington's disease, 13.1
Hyaline membrane disease, **20.8**
Hyperaldosteronism, 3.11, 11.6
Hypercalcemia, **3.15**
Hyperemesis gravidarum, 18.4
Hyperkalemia, 3.11, **3.12**
Hypermetropia, 14.1
Hypersomnia, 13.6
Hypertension, **4.3**
Hyperthyroidism, **11.9**
Hypnotic drugs, **23.17**
Hypoaldosteronism, 3.11

Hypocalcemia, **3.16**
Hypochondriasis, 22.11
Hypoglycemia, 11.11
Hypokalemia, 3.11, **3.13**
Hypothyroidism, **11.10**

Ibuprofen, 23.4
IDDM, 11.11
Identification, 22.2
Ileus, 6.26
Illusions, 22.3
Immunizations, **21.7**
Incubation period, **21.6**
Inderal, 23.1
Indomethacin, 23.4
Infectious mononucleosis, 21.5, 21.6
Infertility, **17.3**
Inflammatory bowel disease, 6.21, **6.25**
Influenza, 5.6, 5.7
Insect stings, 16.15
Insomnia, 13.6
Insulin, 11.1, **11.12**
Intestinal infarction, 6.21
Intestinal injury, 16.5
Intestinal obstruction, 6.21, **6.26**
Intracranial pressure, **13.8**
Introjection, 22.2
Intropin, 23.1
Intussusception, **20.18**
IQ tests, **19.4**
Iron deficiency, 10.4
Isoniazid, 23.3
Isordil, 23.1
Isosorbide dinitrate, 23.7
Isotonic, 3.17
IV calculation, **2.13**
IV solutions, **3.17**

Janeway spots, 9.2
Jaundice, 6.10
Jaundice, **6.12**
Jaundice, neonatal, **20.9**
Juvenile rheumatoid arthritis, **21.15**

Kaposi sarcoma, 8.3
Keflex, 23.1

Kernicterus, 20.9
Kernig's sign, 9.2
Ketoacidosis, 11.11
Ketones, 7.2
Kidneys, **7.5**
Kidney injury, 16.6
Kidney stones, **7.4**
Kidney transplantation, **7.9**
Klumpke paralysis, 20.1
Köbner phenomenon, 15.5
Koplik's spots, 6.2, 9.2
Korsakoff encephalopathy, 2.11, 22.4
Kussmaul respiration, 5.2
Kussmaul's sign, 4.2

Labor, **18.12**, **18.13**, **18.14**
Lactase deficiency, 6.19
Lanoxin, 23.1
Large for gestational age, **20.5**
Laryngotracheobronchitis, 21.9
Lasix, 23.1
L-asparaginase, 23.22
Late decelerations, 18.11
LDL, 4.4
Leukemia, **10.7**, **10.8**
Leukemia, **21.17**
Leukocytosis, 10.2
Leukopenia, 10.2
Levodopa, 23.21
LH, 11.2
Librium, 23.1
Lidocaine, 23.1
Lipitor, 23.1
Lithium, **23.19**
Lithium toxicity, 22.13
Liver, **6.10**, **6.11**, **6.12**, **6.13**, **6.14**, **6.15**
Liver cirrhosis, **6.14**
Liver injury, 16.5
Loop diuretics, 23.8
LSD, 22.15
Lung cancer, **5.15**
Lung sounds, **5.3**
Lupus, **12.7**
Lupus, drug-induced, 23.2
Lymphocytes, 9.3
Lymphoma, **10.10**

Maalox, 23.1
Magnesium sulfate, 23.15
Major depression, **22.12**
Malabsorption, 6.19
Maldigestion, 6.19
Malignant melanoma,15.8
Malingering, 22.11
Mammography, 1.8
Manipulation, 22.1
Mannitol, 23.8
MAO inhibitors, 23.18
Marasmus, 6.1
Maslow's hierarchy, **1.5**
Mastectomy, 17.13
Mastitis, **18.23**
Mastoid ecchymosis, 16.3
McBurney's sign, 9.2
Measles, 21.5, 21.6
Melena, 6.3, 6.7
Mellaril, 23.1
Ménière's disease, **14.11**
Meningitis, **13.9**
Menopause, **17.10**
Menstrual cycle, **17.1**
Menstruation, 17.1, **17.4**
Mental retardation, 19.4
Mental status, **22.4**
Metric system, **24.1**
Migraine, 13.7
Miosis, 13.4
Mitral regurgitation, 4.20
Mitral stenosis, 4.20
Mitral valve prolapse, 4.20
Monistat, 23.1
Moon face, 11.5
Moro reflex, 20.4
Motor development, **19.2**
Motrin, 23.1
Mouth, **6.2**
Multiple myeloma, **10.9**
Multiple sclerosis, **13.14**
Mumps, 21.5, 21.6
Murphy's sign, 6.16, 9.2
Mycoplasma, 5.7
Mydriasis, 13.4
Myocardial infarction, 4.5, **4.8**

Myocardial infarction, complications, **4.9**
Myocarditis, **4.18**
Myopia, 14.1
Myxedema, 11.10

Nägele's rule, 18.5
NANDA, 1.4
Narcissistic personality, 22.9
Narcolepsy, 13.6, 13.17
Nasal flaring, 5.2
Nearsightedness, 14.1
Nembutal, 23.1
Neologisms, 22.4
Nephritic syndrome, 7.6
Nephrotic syndrome, 7.6
Nerve injuries, **16.9**
Neuroleptics, **23.20**
Neutrophils, 9.3
NIDDM, 11.11
Nifedipine, 23.6
Nipple discharge, **17.11**
Nitrates, **23.7**
Nitroglycerin, 23.7
Nitrostat, 23.1
Nonstress test, 18.10
Nosocomial infections, **9.4**
NSAIDs, **23.4**
Nulligravida, 18.1
Nullipara, 18.1
Nursing diagnoses, **1.4**
Nursing process, **1.3**
Nutrition, **6.1**
Nutrition, newborn, **19.1**

Obesity, 6.1
Obsessive personality, 22.9, 22.10
Obstetrics, drugs for, **23.15**
Omeprazole, 23.13
Oncovin, 23.1
On-off phenomenon, 13.13
Opioids, 22.15
Opisthotonus, 9.2
Oral contraceptives, 23.14
Orthopnea, 4.2
Ortolani test, 20.20
Osler's nodes, 9.2

Osmolarity, 3.17
Osmosis, **3.1**
Osteoarthritis, 12.2, **12.3**
Osteomyelitis, **12.11**
Osteoporosis, **12.8**
Otitis media, **21.11**
Otosclerosis, **14.9**
Ototoxicity, 23.2
Ounce, 24.2
Ovarian cancer, **17.16**
Overhydration, **3.10**
Ovulation, 17.1
Oxygen delivery systems, 5.4
Oxytocin, 23.15

Pacemakers, **4.11**
PACU, 1.12
Palmar erythema, 6.10
Pancreatitis, **6.18**
Pancreatitis, 6.4
Panic attack, 22.10
Pap smear, 1.8
Paranoia, 22.1, 22.9
Paraplegia, **13.11**
Parathormone, 5.15, 11.1
Parity, **18.1**
Parkinson's disease, **13.13**, **23.21**
Parkinsonism, 23.20
Passive-aggressive personality, 22.9
Patent ductus arteriosus, 20.13
PEEP, 5.14
Pelvic inflammatory disease, **17.9**
Penicillins, 23.3
PenVee, 23.1
Peptic ulcer, 4.6, 6.4, **6.9**, **23.13**
Pericarditis, **4.16**
Peripheral neuropathies, **13.12**
Peritoneal dialysis, 7.8
Peritonitis, **6.27**, 16.5
Pernicious anemia, 6.8, 10.4
Personality disorders, **22.9**
Pertussis, 21.5, 21.6
Phantom pain, 12.12
Phenothiazines, 23.20
Phenylbutazone, 23.4
Phenytoin, 23.11

Phlebothrombosis, 4.23, **4.28**
Phobia, 22.10
Photosensitivity, 23.2
Phototherapy, 20.9
Piaget, 19.3
Pint, 24.3
Pitocin, 23.1
Pituitary, **11.1**
Pituitary hyperfunction, **11.3**
Pituitary hypofunction, **11.2**
Placenta previa, 18.13
Platelet defects, 10.11
Platinol, 23.1
Pleurisy, 4.6
Pneumoconiosis, 5.13
Pneumocystis jirovecii, 5.7, 8.3
Pneumonia, **5.7**
Pneumonitis, 5.13
Pneumothorax, 4.6, **5.5**, 16.4
Pneumovax, 5.7
Poisoning, **16.2**
Polio, 21.7
Polyarteritis nodosa, 4.27
Polycystic ovaries 17.5
Postmaturity, **20.7**
Postoperative care, **1.12**
Postpartum hemorrhage, **18.21**
Posttraumatic stress disorder, 22.10
Potassium levels, **3.11**
Pott's fracture, 16.7
Preeclampsia, 18.4
Preeclampsia, **18.8**
Pregnancy, problems, **18.3**
Pregnancy, signs of, **18.2**
Pregnancy, signs of danger, **18.4**
Pregnancy test, 17.2
Premature labor, 18.6, **18.17**
Prematurity, **20.6**
Preoperative care, **1.11**
Presbyacusis, **14.10**
Presbyopia, 14.1
Prescriptions, **24.5**
Prilosec, 23.1
Primigravida, 18.1
Primipara, 18.1
Prinzmetal angina, 4.5

Procainamide, 23.11
Procardia, 23.1
Progesterone, 11.1, 23.14
Projection, 22.2
Prolactin, 11.1, 11.3
Prolixin, 23.1
Prone position, 1.7, 21.2
Pronestyl, 23.1
Propanolol, 23.6
Prostaglandin E_2, 23.15
Prostate cancer, **7.11**
Prostate hypertrophy, **7.10**
Prostin E2, 23.1
Proton pump inhibitors, 23.13
Proventil, 23.1
Prozac, 23.1, 23.18
Psoriasis, **15.5**
Psychological development, **19.3**
PTH, 5.15, 11.1
Puerperal infection, **18.22**
Pulmonary care principles, **5.4**
Pulmonary embolism, 4.6
Pulmonary fibrosis, 5.13
Pulse, 1.10
Pulsus alternans, 4.2
Pulsus paradoxus, 4.2
PUVA therapy, 15.5
Pyloric stenosis, **20.17**

Quadriplegia, **13.11**
Quart, 24.3
Quickening, 18.2
Quincke sign, 4.20
Quinidine, 23.11

Radiotherapy, 1.9
Rationalization, 22.2
Raynaud's phenomenon, 4.23, **4.25**
Reaction formation, 22.2
Red blood cells, **10.3**
Reflexes, **20.4**
Refraction, **14.1**
Regional enteritis, **6.25**
Regression, 22.2
Reiter's syndrome, 12.6
Renal failure, acute, **7.7**

Renal failure, chronic, **7.8**
Renal toxicity, 23.2
Renin, 7.1
Repression, 22.2
Residual volume, 4.28
Respiration, 1.10
Respiratory distress syndrome, **20.8**
Respiratory tract infections, 9.4, **21.8**
Restrictive lung diseases, **5.13**
Retina detachment, **14.7**
Retinoic acid, 15.3
Retinoids, 20.11
Reverse isolation technique, 1.9
Reye's syndrome, **21.13**, 23.4
Rheumatic fever, 4.19, **21.14**
Rheumatic heart disease, **4.19**
Rheumatoid arthritis, 12.2, **12.4**
Rickets, 2.11
Rifampin, 23.3
Rolaids, 23.1
Roseola, 21.5
Roth spots, 9.2
Rubella, 21.5
Rubeola, 21.5

Sabin, 21.7
Salicylate intoxication, 23.4
Salk, 21.7
Scarlet fever, 21.5, 21.6
Schilling test, 10.4
Schizoid personality, 22.9
Schizophrenia, **22.14**
Scurvy, 2.11
Seborrheic eczema, **15.4**
Seborrheic keratosis,15.8
Seconal, 23.1
Sengstaken tube, 6.7
Sepsis, 9.4
Sepsis, neonatal, **20.10**
Sex hormones, **23.14**
Sexually transmitted diseases, **8.1**
Sheehan's syndrome, 11.2
Shock lung, **5.14**
Shock, **4.14**, **4.15**
Sickle cell anemia, 10.4
Side-effects, **23.2**

Sigmoidoscopy, 1.8
Sims position, 1.7
Sinemet, 23.1
Sinus node, 4.1
Sinusitis, 5.6
Skin integrity, 1.4
Skin lesions, **15.1**
Skin tumors, **15.8**
Sleep apnea, 13.6
Sleep disorders, **13.6**
Small for gestational age, **20.5**
Smoking, 2.1
Social isolation, 1.4
Sodium levels, **3.8**
Somatization, 22.1, **22.11**
Specific gravity, 7.2
Spider angioma, 6.10
Spider bites, 16.15
Spina bifida, 20.12
Spinnbarkeit, 17.1
Spironolactone, 23.8
Spleen rupture, 16.5
Splenomegaly, 6.10
Spondyloarthropathies, **12.6**
Sprains, **16.8**
Sprue, 6.19
Stasis dermatitis, **15.6**
Stein-Leventhal syndrome, 17.5
Strawberry tongue, 6.2
Strep throat, 5.6
Streptokinase, 23.10
Streptomycin, 23.1
Stress test, 18.10
Stridor, 5.3
Stroke, **13.10**
Stye, 14.5
Subarachnoid hemorrhage, 13.7
Subdural hematoma, 16.3
Suicide, 22.1
Sulfonamides, 23.3
Sulfonylureas, **11.13**
Supine position, 1.7, 21.2
Surfactant, 20.8
Swan neck deformity, 12.1, 12.2
Sympathetic nerves, 4.1
Syphilis, 8.1

Systemic lupus erythematosus, **12.7**

Tagamet, 23.1
Tamoxifen, 17.13
Tamponade, **4.17**, 16.4
Tardive dyskinesia, 22.14, 23.20
Temperature, 1.10, **24.4**
Teratogens, **20.11**
Terbutaline, 23.12, 23.15
Testicular feminization, 17.5
Testosterone, 11.1
Tetracyclines, 23.3
Tetrex, 23.1
Thalassemia, 10.4
Thalidomide, 20.11
Theo-Dur, 23.1
Theophylline, 23.12
Thiazides, 23.8
Thorazine, 23.1
Thought process, 22.4
Thrombocytopenia, 10.2, **10.12**
Thrombophlebitis, 4.23
Thrush, 6.2
TIA, 13.10
Tinnitus, 14.8
Tissue perfusion, 1.4
Tofranil, 23.1
Tonsillitis, 5.6, **21.12**
Tophi, 12.1
Tracheitis, 21.8
Traction, **16.11**
Trademarks, **23.1**
Transfusion reactions, **10.6**
Transfusion risks, 10.5
Transient ischemic attack, 13.10
Traube sign, 4.20
Trauma, **16.1**
Trendelenburg position, 1.7
Tricor, 23.1
Tricyclic antidepressants, 23.18
Trisomy 21, **20.15**
Trousseau sign, 3.17, 4.28
TSH, 11.2
Tuberculin skin test, 5.8
Tuberculosis, **5.8**
Tums, 23.1

Turner syndrome, 17.5
Tylenol, 23.1
Tyramine, 23.18
Ulcerative colitis, 6.25
Undoing, 22.2
Universal precautions, 1.6
Upper respiratory infections, 5.6
Urethra rupture
Urethritis, 7.3
Uric acid, 7.5
Urinary elimination, 1.4
Urinary tract infections, 7.3, 9.4
Urine, 7.2
Urine collection, 7.5
Urokinase, 23.10
Uterine myomas, 17.18
Uterus rupture, 18.13

Vagus nerve, 4.1
Valium, 23.1
Varicella, 21.5
Varicose veins, 15.7
Vasculitis, 4.27
Ventricular flutter, 4.10
Venturi mask, 5.4
Vertigo, 14.11
Vincristine, 23.22
Violence, 1.4, 22.1
Vital capacity, 4.28
Vital signs, 1.10
Vital signs, newborn, 20.3
Vitamins, 2.11
Volkmann's contracture, 16.7
von Willebrand's disease, 10.13

Warfarin, 20.11, 23.10
Wernicke encephalopathy, 2.11, 22.3
Wheezing, 5.3
Wilms' tumor, 21.18
Wound care, 1.13
Wound infections, 9.4
Xanthomas, 6.10
Xylocaine, 23.1
Zantac, 23.1
Zidovudine, 8.3
Zocor, 23.1

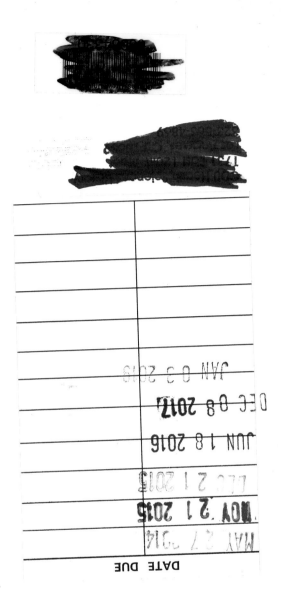